Renal Diet Cookbook For Beginners

Quick and Easy Low Sodium Recipes. Stop Kidney Disease and Avoid Dialysis

Beryl Ramirez

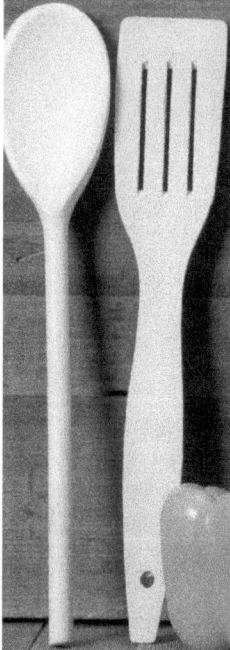

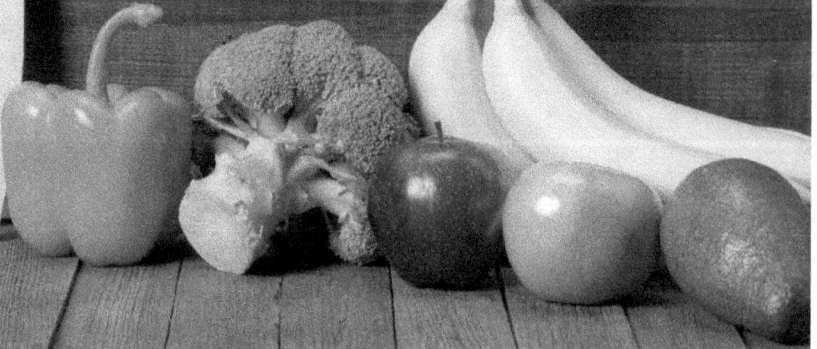

Table of Content

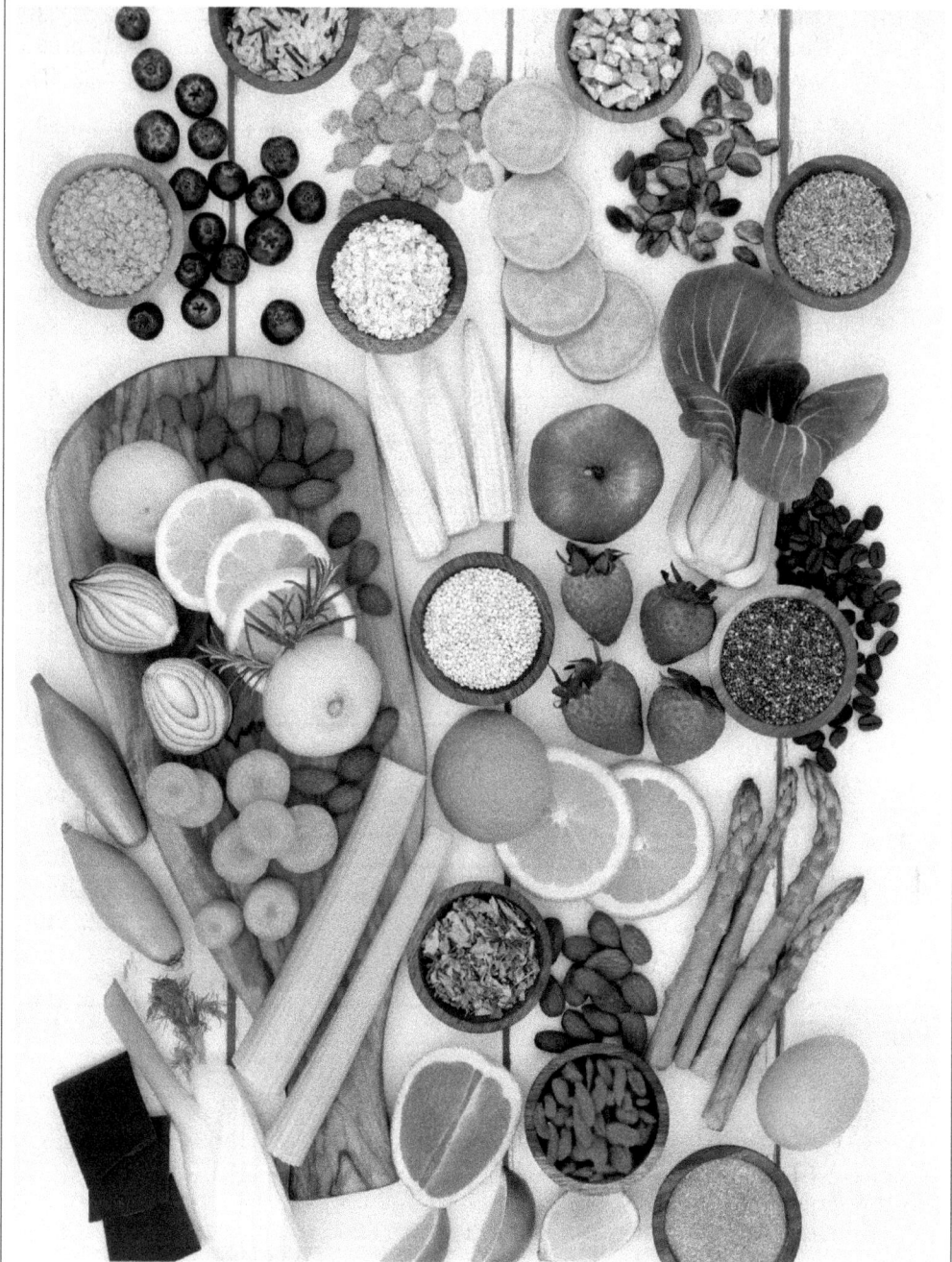

INTRODUCTION

Changing your diet is not as limiting as you think: many whole foods can easily replace refined, processed foods all too common in everyday meals. Many simple snacks and easy foods to eat on the go can fit well into a renal diet. It's a culinary journey that can boost your body's vital functions, in addition to improving your kidneys by reducing the amount of waste produced. Diet is one of the most important factors in our health. What we eat today determines how well we live and function tomorrow. When we have a choice at a better life, despite the challenges of renal failure, it's crucial to take action as soon as possible to ensure we have the best opportunity to live life to the fullest and make the most of our choices.

The renal diet focuses primarily on supporting kidney health but in doing so, you'll improve many other aspects of your health, as well. It can also be customized to fit all levels of kidney disease, from early stages and minor infections to more significant renal impairment and dialysis. Preventing the later stages is the main goal, though reaching this stage can still be treated with careful consideration of your dietary choices. In addition to medical treatment, the diet provides a way for you to gain control over your health and progression. It can mean the difference between a complete renal failure or a manageable chronic condition, where you can lead a regular, enjoyable life despite having kidney issues.

Whether or not the medication is a part of your treatment plan, your diet takes on a significant role in the health of your kidneys. Some herbs and vitamins can boost the medicinal properties found in foods and give your kidneys additional support, while limiting other ingredients which, in excess, can lead to complete renal failure if there are already signs of kidney impairment.

Thanks to this cookbook you will discover numerous recipes that will help you take care of your kidneys and have a healthy lifestyle

Understanding Kidney Disease

The human kidneys are a pair of bean-shaped organs that are located at the base of the rib cage. The main function of the kidneys is to filter out waste products, excess fluids, and other impurities of the blood. These are normally stored in the bladder and excreted during urination. Other functions of the kidneys include:

- Regulating pH, sodium, and potassium levels in the body.

- Producing hormones that maintain normal flow of the blood.

- Stimulating hormones that control the production of erythrocytes or red blood cells.

- Activating a form of Vitamin D that aids in calcium absorption.

Like any major organ of the body, kidneys can get damaged if not maintained properly. According to the National Kidney Foundation, kidney disease affects almost 26 million American adults. Kidney disease happens when your kidneys are damaged and hence, not functioning well. This damage may be caused by different chronic diseases such as diabetes, hypertension, and cardiovascular diseases. If not managed well, kidney disease can lead to serious complications such as bone diseases, nerve damage, and malnutrition. When your kidneys stop working completely, your nephrologist may require you to undergo dialysis treatment. Also referred to as renal replacement therapy, dialysis is the process of filtering and purifying the blood using a machine. A dialysis treatment can not cure kidney disease, but it can prolong a person's life.

Different Types of Kidney Disease

The following are the different types of kidney disease:

Chronic Kidney Disease (CKD)

This is the most common form of kidney disease in humans. Chronic Kidney Disease (CKD) is a long-term, progressive condition that can affect anyone – young or old. The most common cause of CKD is hypertension or high blood pressure. Hypertension can increase the pressure on the glomeruli, the tiny blood vessels in the kidneys that filtrate the blood. It is extremely harmful to the kidneys and can lead to impaired kidney function over time. When the kidneys are no longer functioning, dialysis is needed to filter wastes and extra fluids out of the blood. If the condition worsens, a kidney transplant may be needed.

Another major cause of CKD is diabetes, a group of diseases that results in abnormal (usually high) blood sugar levels. This is extremely harmful because it damages the blood vessels of the kidneys. Damaged blood vessels can impair the main function of the kidneys – filtering out wastes in the blood. When your body becomes loaded with so many wastes, kidney failure is more likely to occur.

Kidney Stones

Kidney stones, also called renal calculi, are solid masses of crystals that originate in the kidneys. This is a common kidney condition that occurs when nutrients and other substances in the blood crystallize and form stones in the kidneys. Kidney stones cause renal colic or severe, excruciating pain on one side of either the back or the abdomen. These stone crystals are normally excreted out of the body during urination.

Glomerulonephritis

It is also called inflammation of the glomeruli, the tiny structures inside the kidney that filter the blood. This disease is commonly caused by drugs, kidney infection, and birth anomalies, or birth defects. Glomerulonephritis is a type of kidney disease that often resolves on its own.

Polycystic Kidney Disease (PKD)

Polycystic kidney disease is an inherited kidney problem that is manifested by the formation of cysts or small sacs of fluid in the kidneys. These cysts interfere with the normal functioning of the kidneys that can lead to kidney failure.

Urinary Tract Infections (UTI)

These are bacterial infections of the upper and lower urinary tract. The most common forms of UTI are infections in the urethra and the bladder. UTI can be easily treated using antibacterial medications and increased fluid intake. But if left untreated, these infections can result in more serious complications, such as kidney failure.

Kidney Failure

Kidney failure is a severe condition that happens when your kidneys lose their ability to filter waste products from your blood. This is also referred to as End-Stage Renal Disease (ESRD) or End-Stage Kidney Disease. When your kidneys stop functioning, it is more likely that you will undergo dialysis treatment or a kidney transplant. Common causes of kidney disease include diabetes, hypertension, autoimmune diseases, nephrotic syndrome, and urinary tract problems.

The following factors can put your kidneys at risk for developing kidney failure:

- Severe dehydration

- Impaired blood supply to the kidneys

- Kidney trauma

- Heart attack

- Urinary tract disorders

- Illegal drug consumption and drug overdose

- Long-term exposure to environmental pollutants

Symptoms of Kidney Failure

People with developing kidney failure are asymptomatic or show no symptoms of the disease during the first few weeks.

However, the following symptoms of kidney failure may start to appear after this period:

- Itching, nausea and vomiting, reduced amounts of urine, muscle cramps, loss of appetite, swelling of the lower extremities (feet and legs).

- Abdominal pain and back pain, shortness of breath, low-grade to high-grade fever, nosebleeds, rashes, excessive drowsiness and easy fatigability, confusion and inability to make decisions, chest pain, anemia, seizures and coma (in severe cases).

If you happen to be experiencing these symptoms, contact your physician immediately.

Stages of Kidney Failure

The following are the five stages of kidney failure:

Stage 1

Stage 1 is referred to as a very mild stage. Patients may be asymptomatic and there is lesser risk for possible complications. Stage 1 can be managed by following a healthy lifestyle. For patients who have diabetes, they need to check their blood sugar levels regularly.

Stage 2

Stage 2 is still classified as a mild form of kidney disease. A person may experience having proteinuria or the presence of protein in the urine. Other physical damages to the kidneys may also be more obvious. A healthy lifestyle and a regular checkup with your doctor are the two most important management practices at this stage.

Stage 3

Stage 3 is already considered a moderate stage of kidney disease. At this stage, the kidneys aren't working as efficiently as before. Symptoms are more visible such as swelling in the upper and lower extremities, and frequent urination. A good lifestyle approach together with some prescribed medications is required during this stage.

Stage 4

Stage 4 is classified as moderate-to-severe-stage of kidney disease. The kidneys are mostly not functioning properly, but it is not yet considered complete kidney failure. Most evident symptoms may include high blood pressure, anemia, and bone disorders. Healthy lifestyle, medications and treatments, together, are the most common forms of management of the disease at this stage.

Stage 5

Stage 5 is considered as the stage of nearly complete or total kidney failure. Different manifestations of the loss of kidney function such as nausea and vomiting, difficulty in breathing, rash, and seizures are more evident. Regular dialysis treatment and kidney transplants are extremely needed at this stage. If not properly managed, this can lead to sudden death.

The severity of kidney damage depends on the glomerular filtration rate (GFR), which is used to evaluate kidney function. Further treatment depends on the severity of chronic kidney disease.

Breakfast

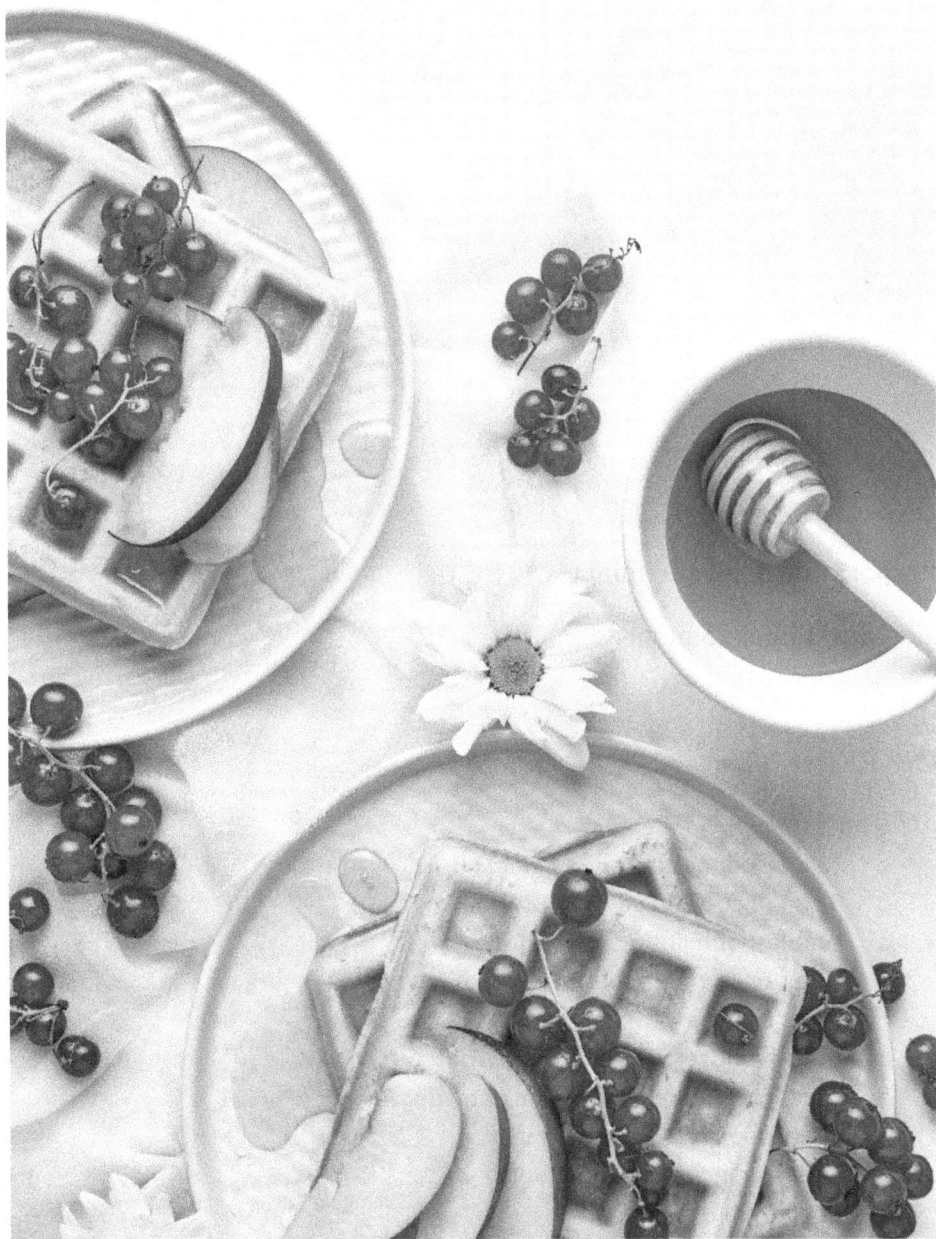

Rhubarb Muffins

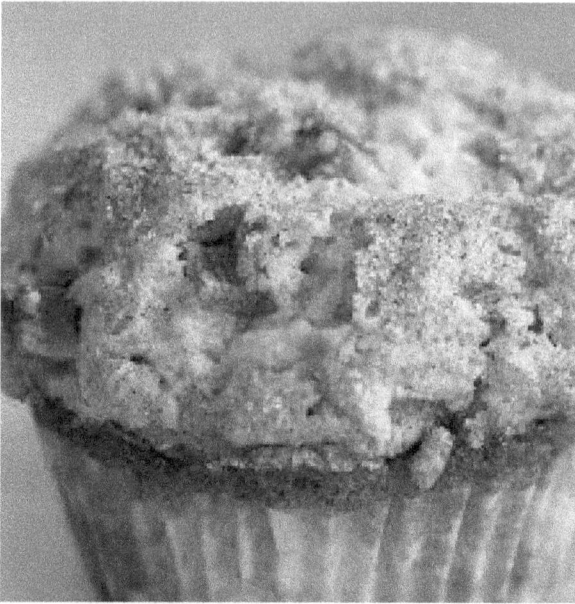

Preparation Time: 10 minutes

Cooking Time: 25 minutes

Serving: 2

INGREDIENTS:

- ○ ½ cup almond meal
- ○ 2 tablespoons crystallized ginger
- ○ ¼ cup of coconut sugar
- ○ 1 tablespoon linseed meal
- ○ ½ cup buckwheat flour
- ○ ¼ cup brown rice flour
- ○ 2 tablespoons powdered arrowroot
- ○ 2 teaspoon gluten-free baking powder
- ○ ½ teaspoon fresh grated ginger
- ○ ½ teaspoon ground cinnamon
- ○ 1 cup rhubarb, sliced
- ○ 1 apple, cored, peeled, and chopped

- o 1/3 cup almond milk, unsweetened
- o ¼ cup olive oil
- o 1 free-range egg
- o 1 teaspoon vanilla extract

DIRECTIONS:

1) In a bowl, mix the almond meal with the crystallized ginger, sugar, linseed meal, buckwheat flour, rice flour, arrowroot powder, grated ginger, baking powder, and cinnamon and stir.
2) In another bowl, mix the rhubarb with the apple, almond milk, oil, egg, and vanilla and stir well. Combine the 2 mixtures, stir well, and divide into a lined muffin tray.
3) Place in the oven at 350 F and bake for 25 minutes.
4) Serve the muffins for breakfast.
5) Enjoy!

NUTRITION (Per Serving): Calories 200; Fat 4; Fiber 6; Phosphorus: 30mg; Potassium: 124mg; Sodium: 20mg; Carbohydrates 13; protein 8.

Buckwheat Granola

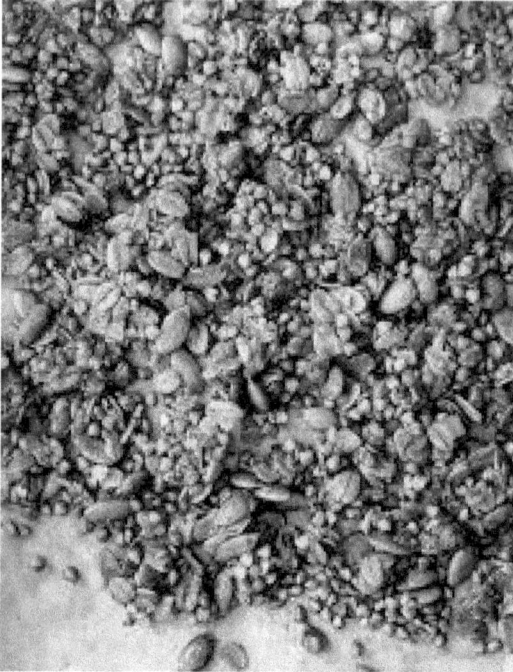

Preparation Time: 10 minutes

Cooking Time: 45 minutes

Serving: 1

INGREDIENTS:

- o   2 cups oats
- o   1 cup buckwheat
- o   1 cup sunflower seeds
- o   1 cup pumpkin seeds
- o   1½ cups dates, pitted and chopped
- o   1 cup apple puree
- o   6 tablespoons coconut oil
- o   5 tablespoons cocoa powder
- o   1 teaspoon fresh grated ginger

DIRECTIONS:

1) In a large bowl, mix the oats with the buckwheat, sunflower seeds, pumpkin seeds, dates, apple puree, oil, cocoa powder, and ginger then stir well.
2) Spread on a lined baking sheet, press well, and place in the oven at 360^0 F for 45 minutes.
3) Leave the granola to cool down, slice, and serve for breakfast.
4) Enjoy!

NUTRITION (Per Serving): Calories 161; Fat 3; Phosphorus: 36mg; Potassium: 14mg; Sodium: 31mg; Fiber 5; Carbs 11; Protein 7.

Mushroom Frittata

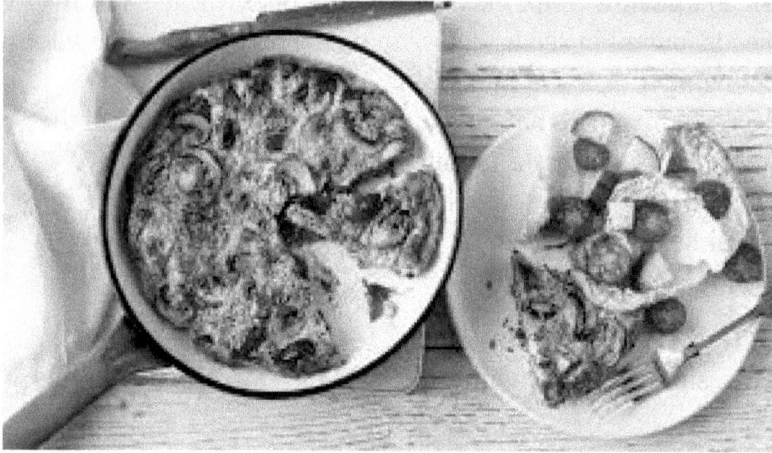

Preparation Time: 10 minutes

Cooking Time: 30 minutes

Serving: 1

INGREDIENTS:

- ¼ cup coconut milk, unsweetened
- 6 eggs
- 1 yellow onion, chopped
- 4 ounces white mushrooms, sliced
- 2 tablespoons olive oil
- 2 cups baby spinach
- A pinch of salt and black pepper

DIRECTIONS:

1) Heat a pan with the oil over medium-high heat, add the onion, stir and cook for 2-3 minutes.
2) Add the mushrooms, salt, and pepper, stir and cook for 2 minutes more.
3) In a bowl, mix the eggs with salt and pepper, stir well and pour over the mushrooms.

4) Add the spinach, mix a bit, place in the oven, and bake at 360 F for 25 minutes.
5) Slice the frittata and serve.
6) Enjoy!

NUTRITION (Per Serving): Calories 200; Fat 3; Phosphorus: 30mg; Potassium: 104mg; Sodium: 13mg; Fiber 6; Carbs 14; Protein 6

Breakfast Crepes

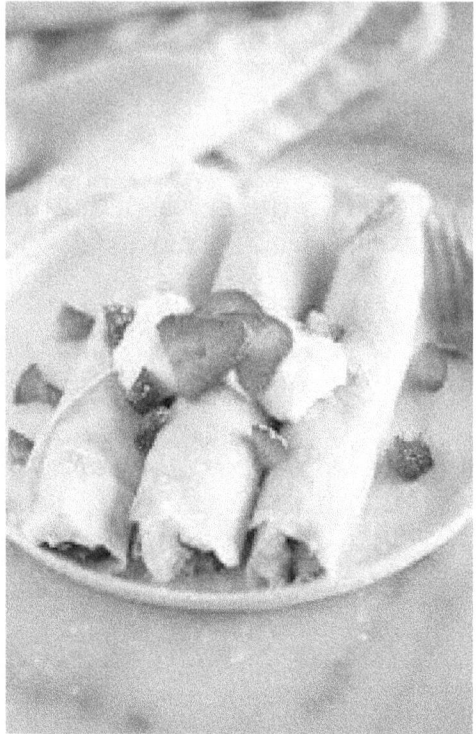

Preparation Time: 10 minutes

Cooking Time: 10 minutes

Serving: 1

INGREDIENTS:

- 2 eggs
- 1 teaspoon vanilla extract
- ½ cup almond milk, unsweetened
- ½ cup water
- 2 tablespoons agave nectar
- 1 cup coconut flour
- 3 tablespoons coconut oil, melted

DIRECTIONS:

1) In a bowl, whisk the eggs with the vanilla extract, almond milk, water, and agave nectar.
2) Add the flour and 2 tablespoons oil gradually and stir until you obtain a smooth batter.
3) Heat a pan with the rest of the oil over medium heat, add some of the batter, spread into the pan, and cook the crepe until it's golden on both sides then transfer to a plate.
4) Repeat with the rest of the batter and serve the crepes.
5) Enjoy!

NUTRITION (Per Serving): Calories 121; Fat 3; Phosphorus: 20mg; Potassium: 94mg; Sodium: 32mg; Fiber 6; Carbs 14; Protein 6

Mushroom Tofu Breakfast

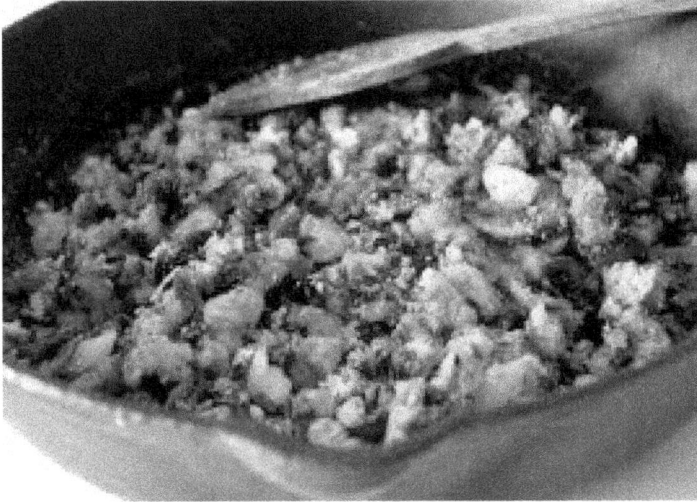

Preparation Time: 10 minutes

Cooking Time: 8-10 minutes

Serving: 2

INGREDIENTS:

- 1 tablespoon of chopped shallots
- ½ cup of sliced white mushrooms
- ⅓ cup medium-firm tofu, crumbled
- ⅓ teaspoon turmeric
- 1 teaspoon of cumin
- ⅓ teaspoon of smoked paprika
- 3 tablespoons of vegetable oil
- Pinch garlic salt
- Pepper

DIRECTIONS:

1) Take a medium saucepan or skillet, add oil. Heat over medium heat.

2) Add shallots, mushrooms, and stir-cook until they become softened for 3-4 minutes.
3) Add tofu, salt, spices, and stir-cook until tofu is tender and cooked well.
4) Serve warm.

NUTRITION (Per Serving): Calories: 217; Fat: 21g; Phosphorus: 77mg; Potassium: 147mg; Sodium: 301mg; Carbohydrates: 3g; Protein: 4g.

Herbed Omelet

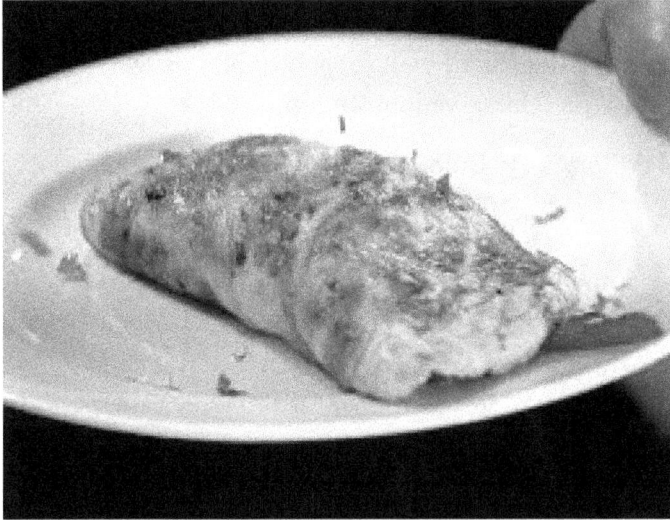

Preparation Time: 5 minutes

Cooking Time: 8-10 minutes

Serving: 2

INGREDIENTS:

- o   4 eggs
- o   2 tablespoons water
- o   1 ½ teaspoons vegetable oil
- o   1 tablespoon chopped onion
- o   ¼ teaspoon basil
- o   ⅛ teaspoon tarragon
- o   ¼ teaspoon parsley (optional)

DIRECTIONS:

1) Take a mixing bowl and beat eggs. Add water and spices; combine.
2) Take a medium saucepan or skillet, add oil. Heat over medium heat.

3) Add onion and stir-cook until become translucent and softened. Set aside.
4) Add the egg mixture in the pan and spread evenly.
5) Cook over both sides until well set and lightly brown.
6) Serve warm with cooked onions on top.

NUTRITION (Per Serving): Calories: 204; Fat: 14g; Phosphorus: 201mg; Potassium: 166mg; Sodium: 174mg; Carbohydrates: 1g; Protein: 14g.

Juice and Smoothies

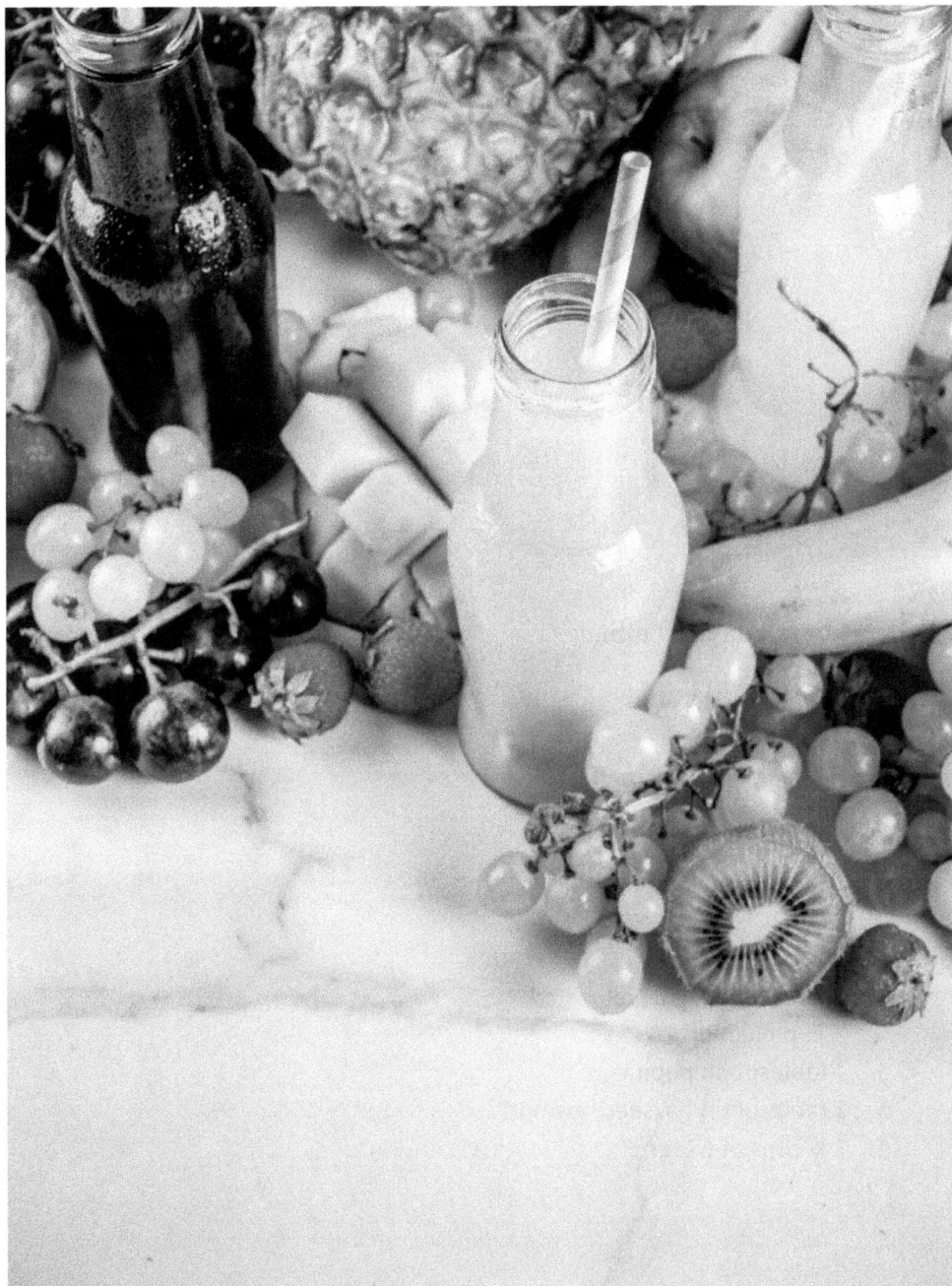

Blueberry and Kale Mix

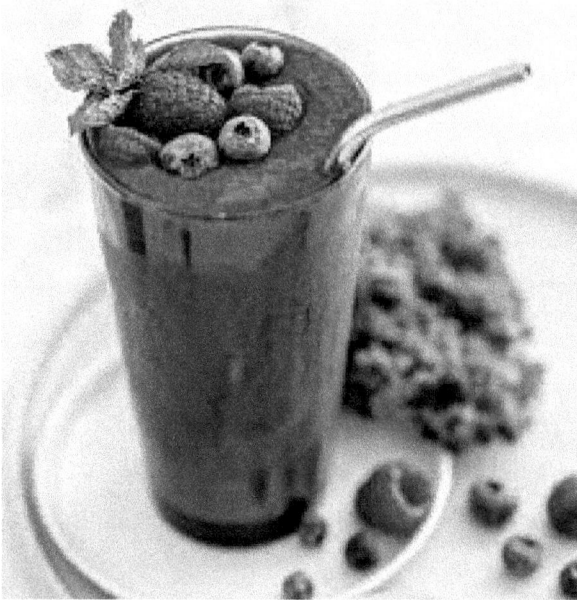

Preparation Time: 10 minutes

Cooking Time: 30 minutes

Serving: 1

INGREDIENTS:

- o ½ cup low-fat Greek Yogurt
- o 1 cup baby kale greens
- o 1 pack stevia
- o 1 tablespoon MCT oil
- o ¼ cup blueberries
- o 1 tablespoon pepitas
- o 1 tablespoon flaxseed, ground
- o 1 ½ cups of water

DIRECTIONS:

1) Add listed ingredients to a blender.
2) Blend until you have a smooth and creamy texture.
3) Serve chilled and enjoy!

NUTRITION (Per Serving): Calories: 307; Fat: 24g; Phosphorus: 36mg; Potassium: 194mg; Sodium: 31mg; Carbohydrates: 14g; Protein: 9g.

Blackberry-Sage Drink

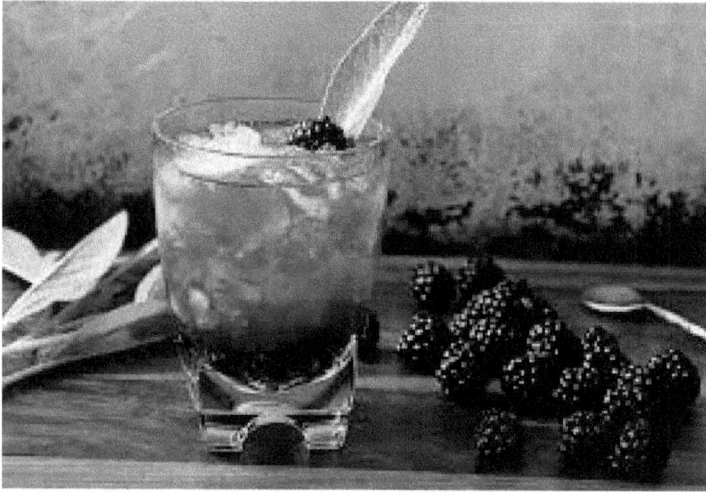

Preparation Time: 10 minutes

Cooking Time: 0 minutes

Serving: 2

INGREDIENTS:

- o 1 cup fresh blackberries
- o 4 sage leaves
- o 10 cups water

DIRECTIONS:

1) Add blackberries, sage leave, and 10 cup water to a blender.
2) Blend well, then strain and refrigerate to chill.
3) Serve.

NUTRITION (Per Serving): Calories: 7; Protein: 0 g; Carbohydrates: 2 g; Cholesterol: 0 mg; Sodium: 7 mg; Potassium: 26 mg; Phosphorus: 3 mg; Calcium: 13 mg; Fiber: 0.7 g.

Pina Colada Spicy Smoothie

Preparation Time: 2 minutes

Cooking Time: 5 minutes

Serving: 2

INGREDIENTS:

- o 1 cup Mascarpone Cheese, firm
- o 1 cup pineapple, canned or fresh
- o 1 teaspoon Stevia or another sweetener
- o ½ cup pineapple juice, unsweetened
- o Pinch red pepper flakes

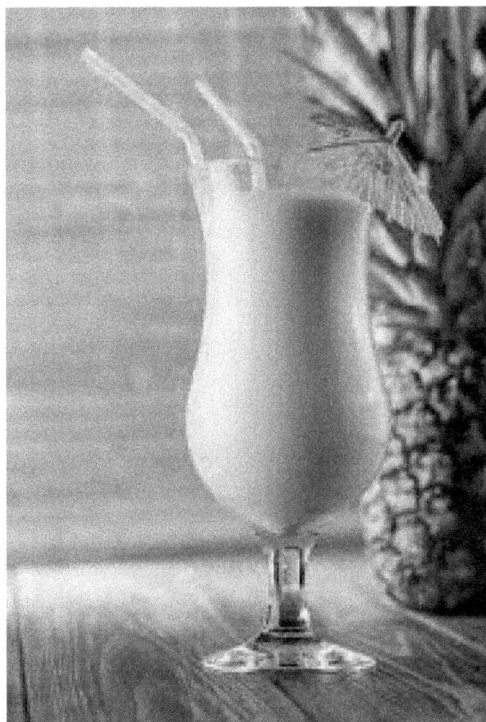

DIRECTIONS:

1) Mix all the ingredients in a blender.
2) Serve.

NUTRITION (Per Serving): Protein - 13.4g; Phosphorus: 23mg; Potassium: 55mg; Sodium: 18mg; Carbohydrates - 32g; Fat - 5g; Calories – 189.

Raspberry Peach Smoothie

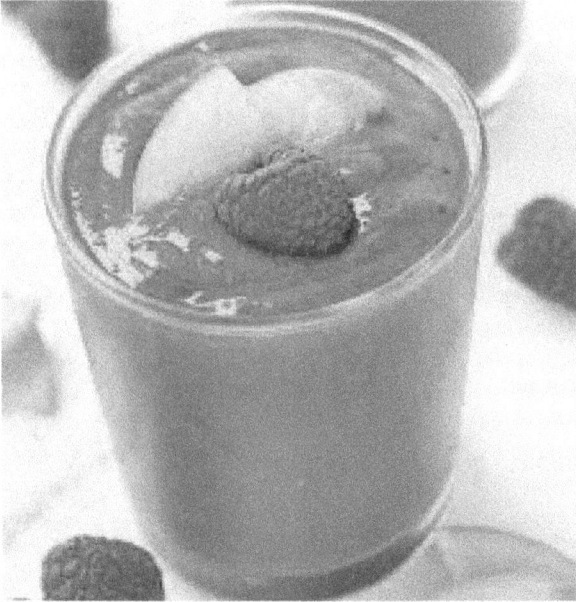

Preparation Time: 5 minutes

Cooking Time: 5 minutes

Serving: 1

INGREDIENTS:

- 1 medium peach, sliced
- 1 cup frozen raspberries
- 1 tablespoon honey
- ½ cup tofu
- 1 cup unfortified almond milk

DIRECTIONS:

1) Mix all the ingredients in your blender.
2) Enjoy!

NUTRITION (Per Serving): Protein - 6.3g; Phosphorus: 29mg; Potassium: 67mg; Sodium: 30mg; Carbohydrates - 23g; Fat - 3.2g; Calories – 129.

Blueberry Smoothie

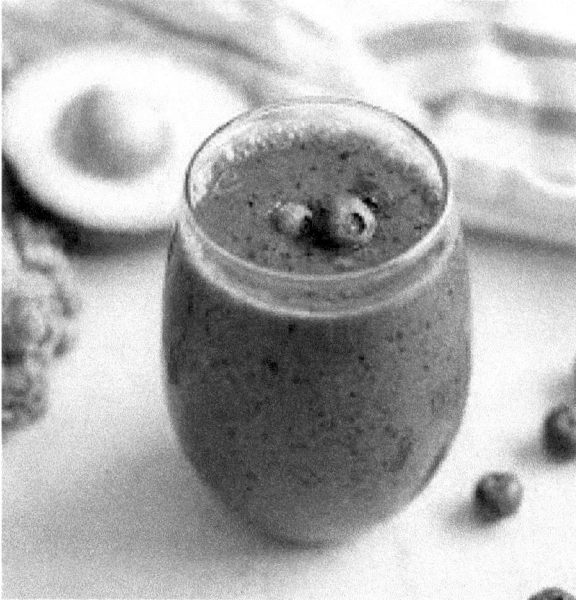

Preparation Time: 5 minutes

Cooking Time: 2 minutes

Serving: 1

INGREDIENTS:

- o   2 cups frozen blueberries (slightly thawed)
- o   1 ¼ cup pineapple juice
- o   2 teaspoon sugar or Splenda
- o   ¾ cup pasteurized egg whites
- o   ½ cup water

DIRECTIONS:

1) Mix all the ingredients in blender, puree and serve.

NUTRITION (Per Serving): Protein - 7.4g; Phosphorus: 36mg; Potassium: 194mg; Sodium: 31mg; Carbohydrates - 31.1g; Fat - 0.75g; Calories - 155.4.

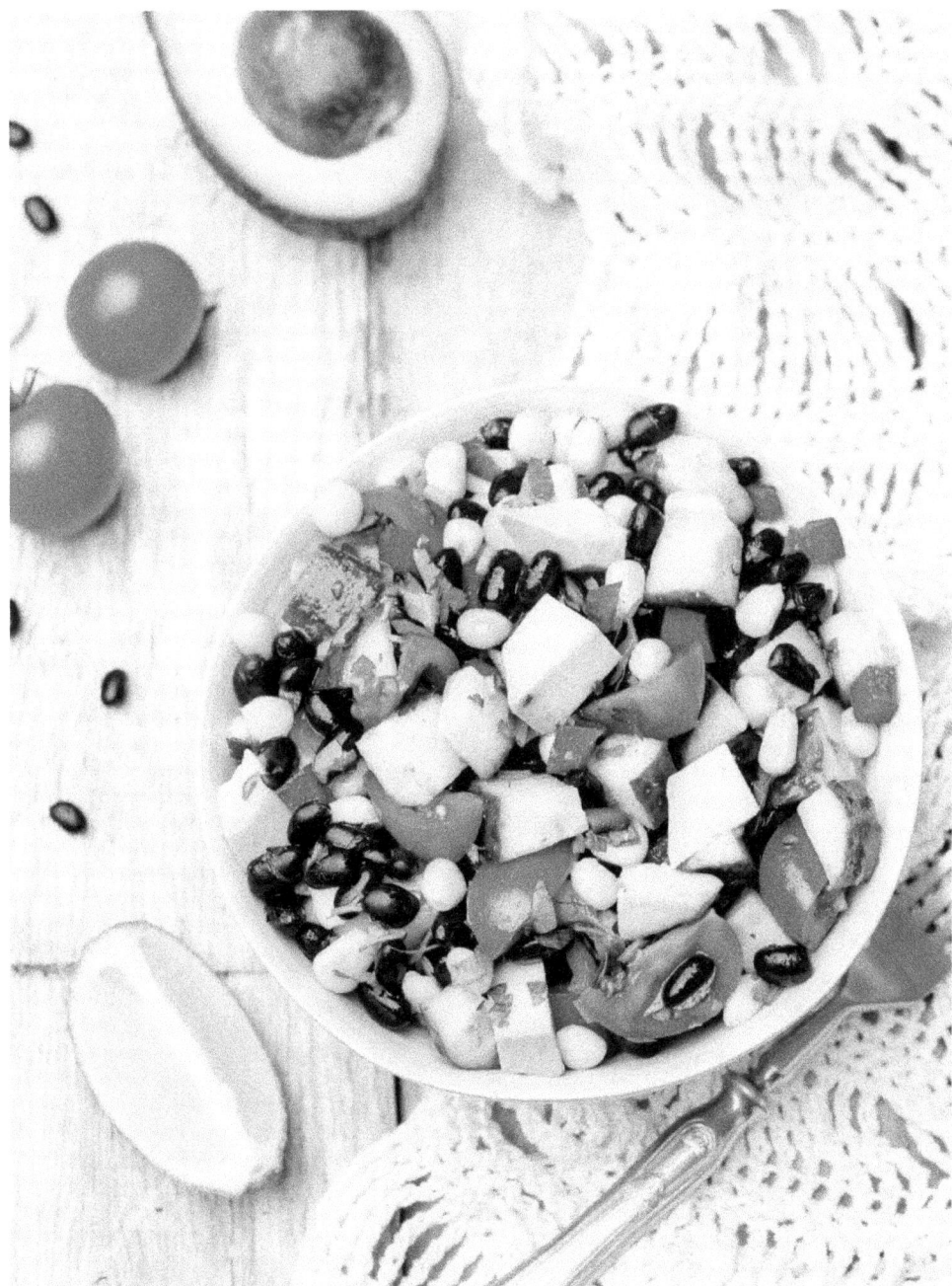

Salads

Broccoli-Cauliflower Salad

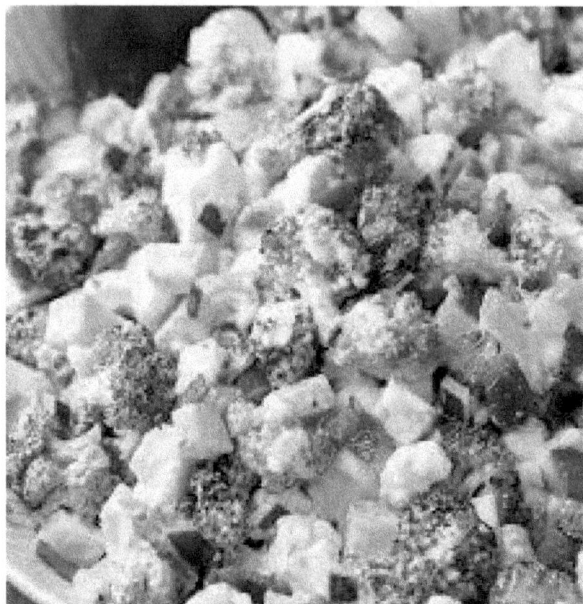

Preparation Time: 5 minutes

Cooking Time: 5 minutes

Serving: 2

INGREDIENTS:

- o   1 tablespoon wine vinegar
- o   1 cup cauliflower florets
- o   ¼ cup white sugar
- o   2 cups hard-cooked eggs
- o   5 slices bacon
- o   1 cup broccoli florets
- o   1 cup cheddar cheese
- o   1 cup mayonnaise

DIRECTIONS:

1) In a bowl add all ingredients and mix well.
2) Serve with dressing.

NUTRITION (Per Serving): Calories 89.8; Fat 4.5 g; Sodium (Na) 51.2 mg; Potassium (K) 257.6 mg; Carbs 11.5 g; Protein 3.0 g; Phosphorus 47 mg.

Cabbage Pear Salad

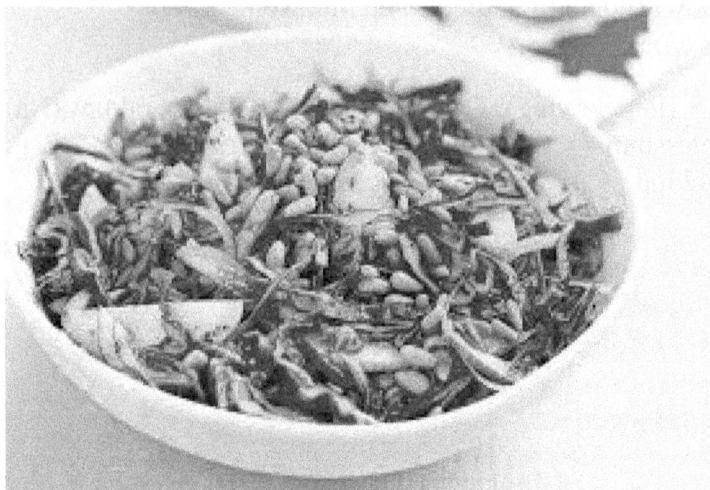

Preparation Time: 10 minutes + 1 hours

Cooking Time: 0 minutes

Serving: 1

INGREDIENTS:

- 2 scallions, chopped
- 2 cups finely shredded green cabbage
- 1 cup finely shredded red cabbage
- ½ red bell pepper, boiled and chopped
- ½ cup chopped cilantro
- 2 celery stalks, chopped
- 1 Asian pear, cored and grated
- ¼ cup olive oil
- Juice of 1 lime
- Zest of 1 lime
- 1 teaspoon granulated sugar

DIRECTIONS:

1) In a mixing bowl, add cabbages, scallions, celery, pear, red pepper, and cilantro. Combine to mix well.
2) Take another mixing bowl; add olive oil, lime juice, lime zest, and sugar. Combine to mix well with each other.
3) Add dressing over and toss well.
4) Refrigerate for 1 hour; serve chilled.

NUTRITION (Per Serving): Calories: 128; Fat: 8g; Phosphorus: 25mg; Potassium: 149mg; Sodium: 57mg; Carbohydrates: 2g; Protein: 6g.

Arugula Parmesan Salad

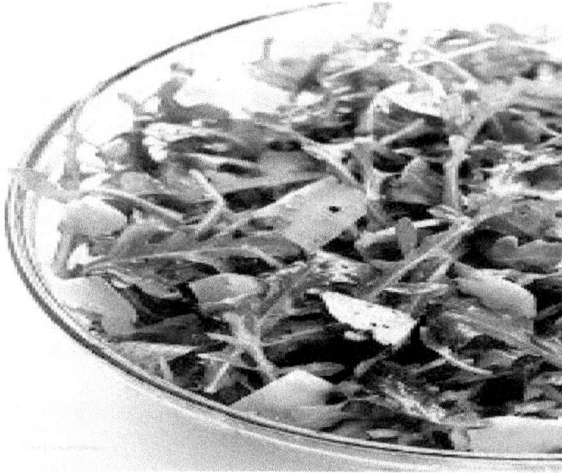

Preparation Time: 10 minutes

Cooking Time: 0 minutes

Serving: 1

INGREDIENTS:

- o 2 cups loosely packed arugula
- o 1 tablespoon extra-virgin olive oil
- o 1 shallot, thinly sliced
- o 3 celery stalks, cut into 1-inch pieces about ¼ inch thick
- o 2 tablespoons white wine vinegar
- o Black pepper (ground), to taste
- o 2 tablespoons Parmesan cheese, grated

DIRECTIONS:

1) In a mixing bowl, add shallot, celery stalks, and arugula. Combine to mix well.
2) Take another mixing bowl; add olive oil, vinegar, and black pepper. Combine to mix well with each other.
3) Add dressing over and toss well.
4) Add cheese on top and serve fresh.

NUTRITION (Per Serving): Calories: 61; Fat: 4g; Phosphorus: 34mg; Potassium: 53mg; Sodium: 55mg; Carbohydrates: 1g; Protein: 2g.

Walnut Salad

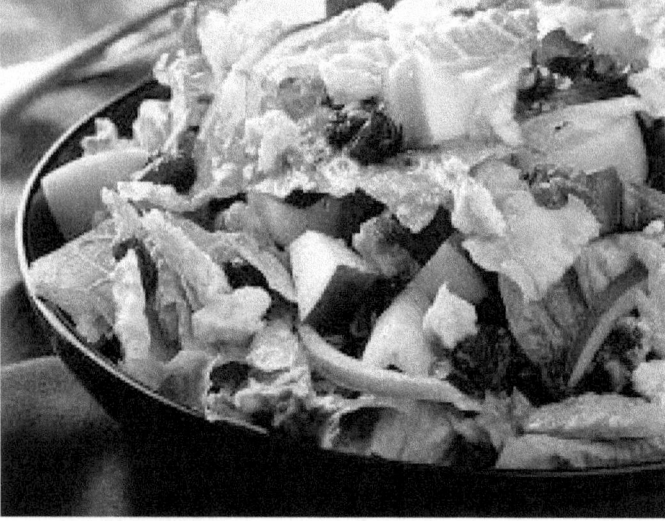

Preparation Time: 7 minutes

Cooking Time: 5 minutes

Serving: 1

INGREDIENTS:

- o 1 oz Feta cheese, crumbled
- o 2 oz walnuts, chopped
- o 1 cup fresh parsley, chopped
- o 1 cup cucumbers, chopped
- o ½ cup tomatoes, chopped
- o ½ red onion, sliced
- o 2 tablespoons sesame oil
- o 1 tablespoon lemon juice
- o 1 teaspoon Italian seasoning

DIRECTIONS:

1) Make the dressing by mixing Italian seasoning, lemon juice, and sesame oil.
2) Then in the salad bowl combine crumbled Feta cheese, walnuts, parsley, cucumbers, tomatoes, and onion.
3) Drizzle the dressing over the salad and mix it up with the help of two spatulas.

NUTRITION (Per Serving): calories 126; fat 11.5; Phosphorus: 40mg; Potassium: 56mg; Sodium: 25mg; fiber 1.5; carbs 4; protein 3.6.

Sliced Figs Salad

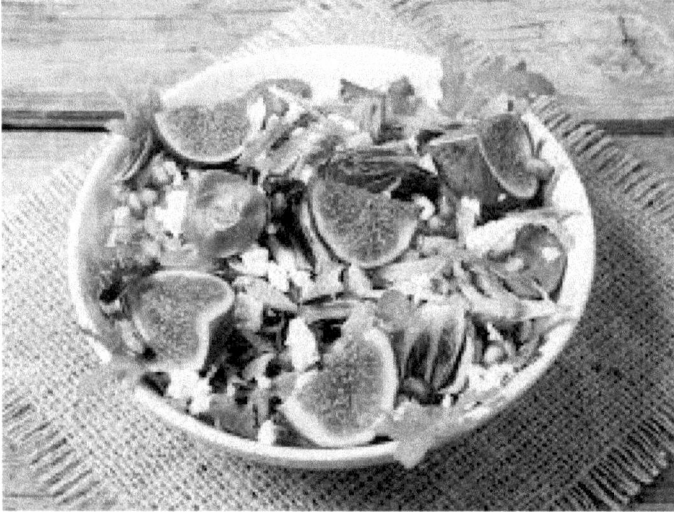

Preparation Time: 10 minutes

Cooking Time: 5 minutes

Serving: 1

INGREDIENTS:

- 1 tablespoon balsamic vinegar
- 1 teaspoon canola oil
- 2 tablespoons almonds, sliced
- 3 figs, sliced
- 2 cups fresh parsley
- 1 cup fresh arugula
- 2 oz Feta cheese, crumbled
- ½ teaspoon salt
- ½ teaspoon honey

DIRECTIONS:

1) Make the salad dressing by mixing balsamic vinegar, canola oil, salt, and honey.
2) Then put sliced almonds and figs in the big bowl.
3) Chop the parsley and add in the fig mixture too.
4) After this, tear arugula.
5) Combine arugula with fig mixture.
6) Add salad dressing and shake the salad well.

NUTRITION (Per Serving): calories 116; fat 6.1; Phosphorus: 45mg; Potassium: 69mg; Sodium: 20mg; fiber 2.8; carbs 13.2; protein 4.1.

Beef Salad

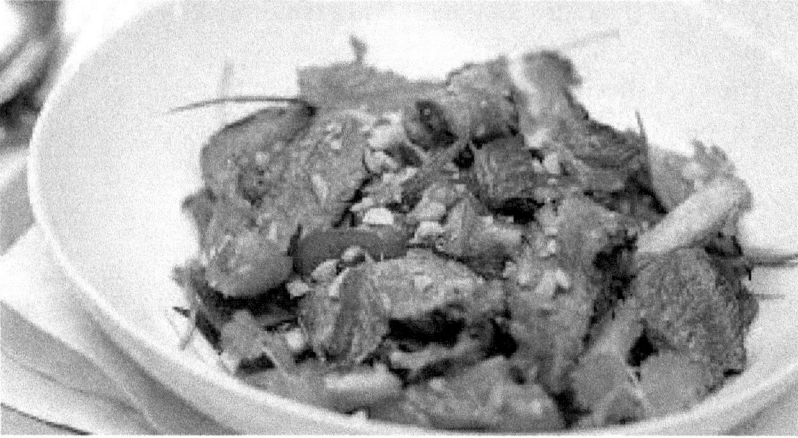

Preparation Time: 15 minutes

Cooking Time: 35 minutes

Serving: 1

INGREDIENTS:

- 8 cups torn romaine lettuce
- ½ cup each julienned cucumber, sweet yellow pepper, and red onion
- 4 teaspoon canola oil
- ½ cup of halved grape tomatoes
- Chili-lime vinaigrette
- ¼ cup fresh lime juice
- 1 teaspoon of grated lime rind
- 1 tablespoon honey
- 1 tablespoon Asian chili sauce
- 2 tablespoon rice vinegar
- 1 tablespoon minced ginger root
- 1 tablespoon fresh lime juice
- 1 tablespoon cornstarch
- 1 teaspoon Asian chili sauce
- 2 cloves garlic, minced

- 1 lb. Beef Strip Loin, Top Sirloin or Flank Steak, thinly sliced

DIRECTIONS:

1) Combine the chili sauce, sesame oil, garlic, lime juice, ginger root, and cornstarch in a medium bowl.
2) Add beef. Toss to coat. Let stand for 10 minutes.
3) In a large frypan, heat 1 teaspoon canola oil.
4) Stir-fry onion, yellow pepper, cucumber, tomatoes until just wilted and hot. Transfer to the clean bowl.
5) Heat the remaining canola oil in the same pan. Stir-fry beef until cooked and browned.
6) Add to wilted vegetables, tossing to combine.
7) Whisk all chili-lime vinaigrette ingredients together.
8) Put chili-lime vinaigrette in the pan. Cook until hot and slightly thickened.
9) Top romaine with veggies and beef and vinaigrette.

NUTRITION (Per Serving): Protein - 13g; Phosphorus: 36mg; Potassium: 194mg; Sodium: 31mg; Carbohydrates - 6g; Fat - 4.3g; Calories – 116

Chicken BBQ Salad

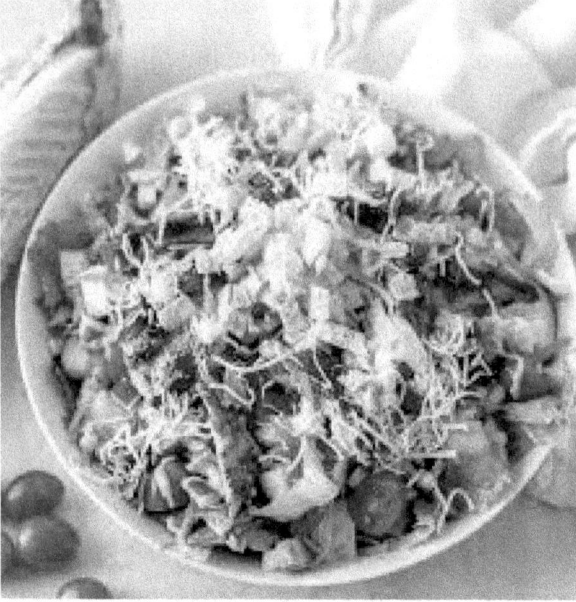

Preparation Time: 10 minutes

Cooking Time: 1 hour and 30 minutes

Serving: 1

INGREDIENTS:

- 1 teaspoon soy sauce
- 4 boneless, skinless chicken breasts
- 2 tablespoon cilantros
- 2 tablespoon extra-virgin olive oil
- 2 cloves garlic
- 1 tablespoon ginger, minced
- 2 yellow peppers, large
- ½ teaspoon hot red chili pepper flakes
- 5 ½ cups mixed salad greens
- 3 tablespoons rice vinegar

DIRECTIONS:

1) Mince fresh cilantro.
2) Whisk together pepper flakes, garlic, ginger, cilantro, and half of the oil in a large bowl.
3) Add chicken breasts and coat well. Cover and refrigerate for 30 minutes.
4) Cut peppers into quarters.
5) Over medium-high heat, grill pepper until they start to blacken, for about fifteen minutes. Remove them to plate.
6) Grill chicken breasts for 15 minutes per side, until done.
7) Chop chicken and warm grilled peppers into ½ inch wide strips. Toss peppers and chicken with remaining vinegar and oil and greens.

NUTRIENTS per **Serving:** Protein - 25g; Phosphorus: 60mg; Potassium: 64mg; Sodium: 31mg; Carbohydrates - 5g; Fat - 5g; Calories – 171.

Soups and Stews

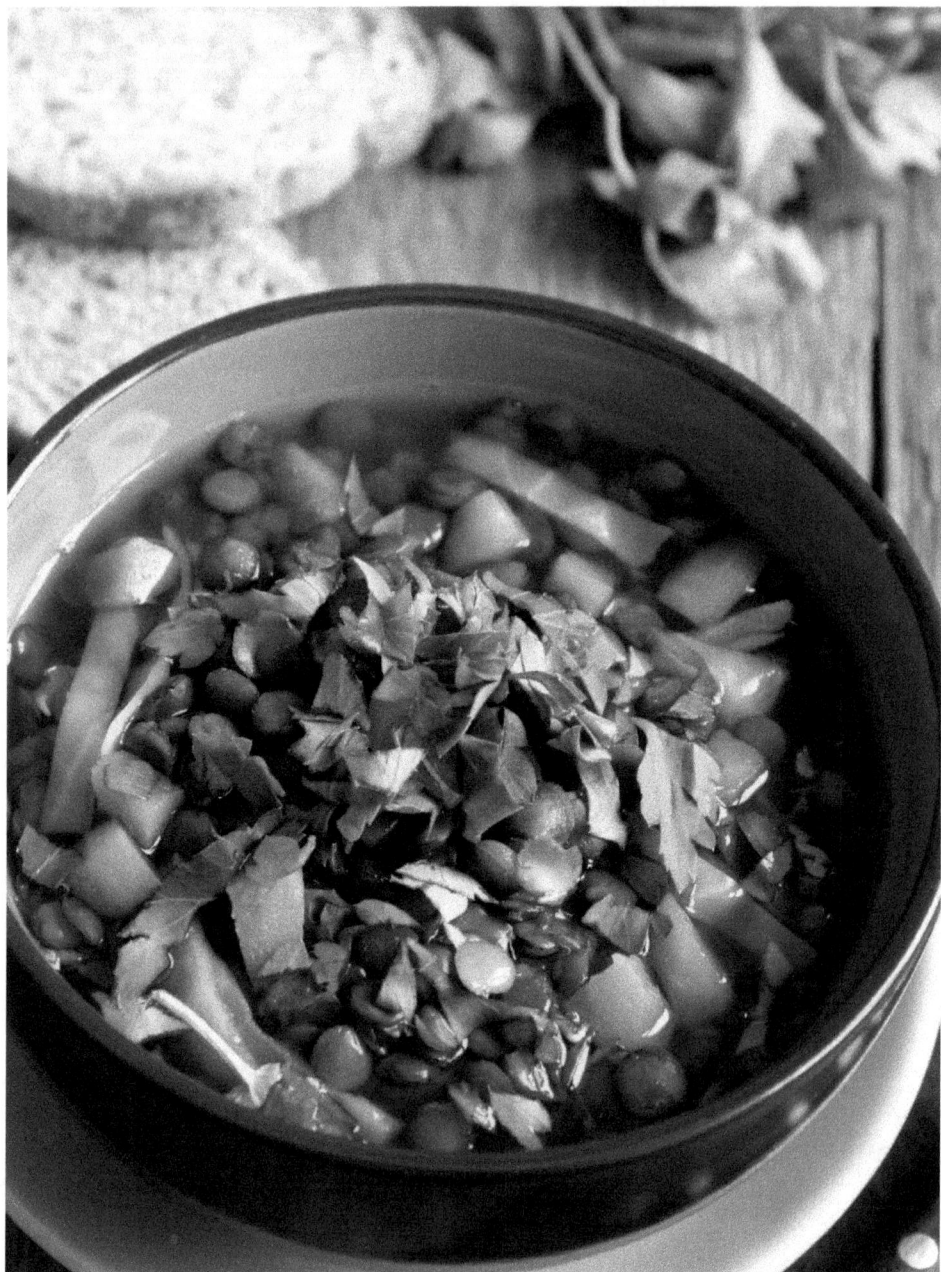

Cabbage Turkey Soup

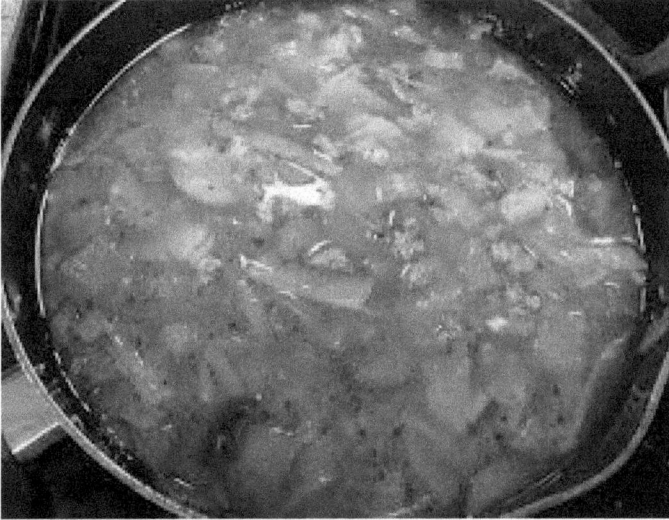

Preparation Time: 10 minutes

Cooking Time: 40-45 minutes

Serving: 1

INGREDIENTS:

- ½ cup shredded green cabbage
- ½ cup bulgur
- 2 dried bay leaves
- 2 tablespoons chopped fresh parsley
- 1 teaspoon chopped fresh sage
- 1 teaspoon chopped fresh thyme
- 1 celery stalk, chopped
- 1 carrot, sliced thin
- ½ sweet onion, chopped
- 1 teaspoon minced garlic
- 1 teaspoon olive oil
- ½ pound cooked ground turkey, 93% lean
- 4 cups of water
- 1 cup chicken stock

- ○ Pinch red pepper flakes
- ○ Black pepper (ground), to taste

DIRECTIONS:

1) Take a large saucepan or cooking pot, add oil. Heat over medium heat.
2) Add turkey and stir-cook for 4-5 minutes until evenly brown.
3) Add onion and garlic and sauté for about 3 minutes to soften veggies.
4) Add water, chicken stock, cabbage, bulgur, celery, carrot, and bay leaves.
5) Boil the mixture.
6) Over low heat, cover, and simmer the mixture for about 30-35 minutes until bulgur is cooked well and tender.
7) Remove bay leaves. Add parsley, sage, thyme, and red pepper flakes; stir mixture and season with black pepper.
8) Serve warm.

NUTRITION (Per Serving): Calories: 83; Fat: 4g; Phosphorus: 91mg; Potassium: 185mg; Sodium: 63mg; Carbohydrates: 2g; Protein: 8g.

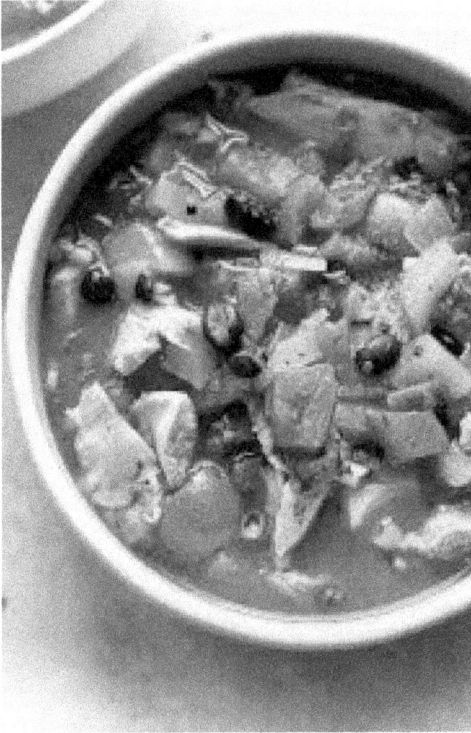

Chicken Fajita Soup

Preparation Time: 10 minutes

Cooking Time: 6 hours 30 minutes

Serving: 2

INGREDIENTS:

o   2 pounds of boneless skinless chicken breasts
o   1 onion chopped
o   1 green pepper chopped
o   3 garlic cloves minced
o   1 tablespoon of butter
o   6 ounces of cream cheese
o   salt and pepper to taste

DIRECTIONS:

1) Add boneless skinless chicken breasts to a slow cooker and cook for 3 hours on high or 6 hours on low in a cup of chicken broth.
2) Season with salt and pepper. When the chicken is done, remove from the slow cooker and shred. (You can strain the leftover broth for the soup.)
3) In a large saucepan fry green pepper, onion, and garlic in 1 tablespoon of butter until they are translucent (2 to 3 minutes).
4) Mash the cream cheese into the veggies with a spoon so that it will combine smoothly as it melts.

NUTRITION (Per Serving): Calories: 306kcal; Carbohydrates: 8.2g; Protein: 26g; Fat: 17g; Saturated Fat: 9g; Cholesterol: 120mg; Sodium: 880mg; Potassium: 757mg; Fiber: 1.6g; Sugar: 3g; Vitamin A: 12.7%; Vitamin C: 26.5%; Calcium: 4.9%; Iron: 4.4%.

Italian Wedding Soup

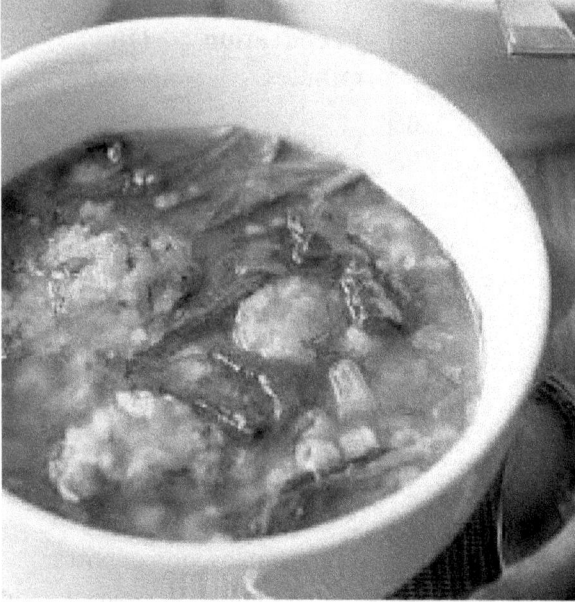

Preparation Time: 15 minutes

Cooking Time: 25 minutes

Serving: 1

INGREDIENTS:

Meatballs:

- o 1 pound of ground beef OR ground pork
- o ½ cup of crushed pork rinds OR almond flour
- o ½ cup of grated Parmesan cheese
- o 1 teaspoon of Italian seasoning
- o ¾ teaspoon of salt
- o ½ teaspoon of pepper
- o 1 large egg

Soup:

- o 2 tablespoons of avocado oil

- ○ ¼ cup of chopped onion
- ○ 4 celery stalks chopped
- ○ 1 teaspoon of salt
- ○ ½ teaspoon of pepper
- ○ 3 cloves garlic minced
- ○ 1 teaspoon of dried oregano
- ○ 6 cups of chicken broth
- ○ 2 cups of riced cauliflower
- ○ Parmesan for sprinkling

DIRECTIONS:

1) Refrigerate until soup is ready.
2) Heat the oil in a large saucepan or stockpot over medium heat until simmering.
3) Add the onion, celery, salt, and pepper and fry until vegetables are soft and tender (about 7 minutes).
4) Add the garlic and cook for 1 minute.
5) Stir in the chicken broth and oregano and simmer for 10 minutes.
6) Add the cauliflower rice and the meatballs and cook for about 5 minutes.
7) Add the spinach leaves and cook until wilted, 2 minutes more. Season to taste.
8) Serve and enjoy.

NUTRITION (Per Serving): Food energy: 303kcal; Total fat: 20.16g; Calories from fat: 181; Cholesterol: 73mg; Carbohydrate: 5.73g; Phosphorus: 36mg; Potassium: 100mg; Sodium: 31mg; Total dietary fiber: 1.86g; Protein: 29.48g.

Cream of Chicken Soup

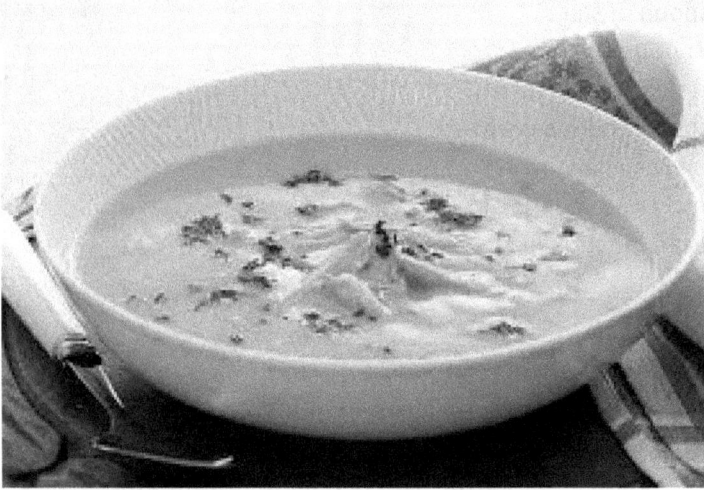

Preparation Time: 10 minutes

Cooking Time: 20 minutes

Serving: 2

INGREDIENTS:

- 2 cups (500 grams) of cauliflower florets
- 2/3 cup (157 ml) of unsweetened original almond milk
- 1 cup (250 ml) of chicken broth
- 1 teaspoon (5 ml) of onion powder
- ½ teaspoon (2.5 ml) of grey sea salt
- ¼ teaspoon (1.23 ml) of garlic powder
- ¼ teaspoon (1.23 ml) of freshly ground black pepper
- 1/8 teaspoon (0.61 ml) of celery seed (optional)
- 1/8 teaspoon (0.61 ml) of dried thyme
- ¼ cup (30 grams) of Beef Gelatin

DIRECTIONS:

1) Place all ingredients, except cooked chicken and gelatin, in a small saucepan.
2) Cover and bring to a boil over medium heat.

3) Turn heat to low and cook for about 7 to 8 minutes, until cauliflower is softened.
4) Remove from the heat.
5) Add around ½ cup of the hot liquid to a medium-sized bowl using a ladle.
6) Add gelatin, one scoop at a time.
7) Stir until dissolved, then add the next scoop.
8) Serve immediately.

NUTRITION (Per Serving): Calories: 198; Calories from Fat: 62.1; Total Fat: 6.9 g Saturated Fat: 1.1 g; Cholesterol: 24 mg; Sodium: 672 mg; Phosphorus: 36mg; Potassium: 194mg; Carbs: 9.4 g; Dietary Fiber: 3.8 g; Net Carbs: 5.6 g; Sugars: 3.3 g; Protein: 26.4 g.

Turkey & Lemon-Grass Soup

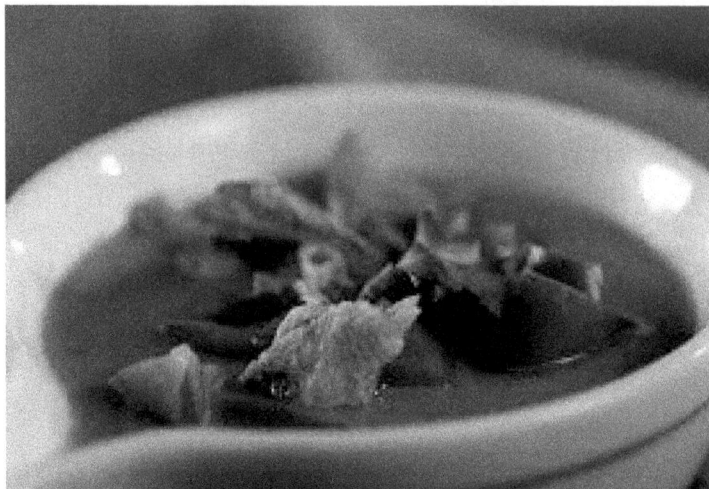

Preparation Time: 5 minutes

Cooking Time: 40 minutes

Serving: 1

INGREDIENTS:

- o 1 fresh lime
- o ¼ cup fresh basil leaves
- o 1 tablespoon cilantro
- o 1 cup canned and drained water chestnuts
- o 1 tablespoon coconut oil
- o 1 thumb-size minced ginger piece
- o 2 chopped scallions
- o 1 finely chopped green chili
- o 4 oz. skinless and sliced turkey breasts
- o 1 minced garlic clove
- o ½ finely sliced stick lemongrass
- o 1 chopped white onion
- o 4 cups of water

DIRECTIONS:

1) Crush the lemongrass, cilantro, chili, 1 tablespoon oil, and basil leaves in a blender or with the help of a pestle and mortar, to form a paste. Keep it aside.
2) Heat a large pan/wok with 1 tablespoon olive oil on high heat.
3) Sauté the onions, garlic, and ginger until soft.
4) Add the turkey and brown each side for 4-5 minutes.
5) Add the broth and stir.
6) Now add the prepared paste and stir.
7) Next, add the water chestnuts, turn down the heat slightly and allow it to simmer for 25-30 minutes or until turkey is thoroughly cooked through.
8) Serve hot with the green onion sprinkled over the top.

NUTRITION (Per Serving): Calories 123; Protein 10 g; Carbs 12 g; Fat 3 g; Sodium (Na) 501 mg; Potassium (K) 151 mg; Phosphorus 110 mg.

Fish and Seafood

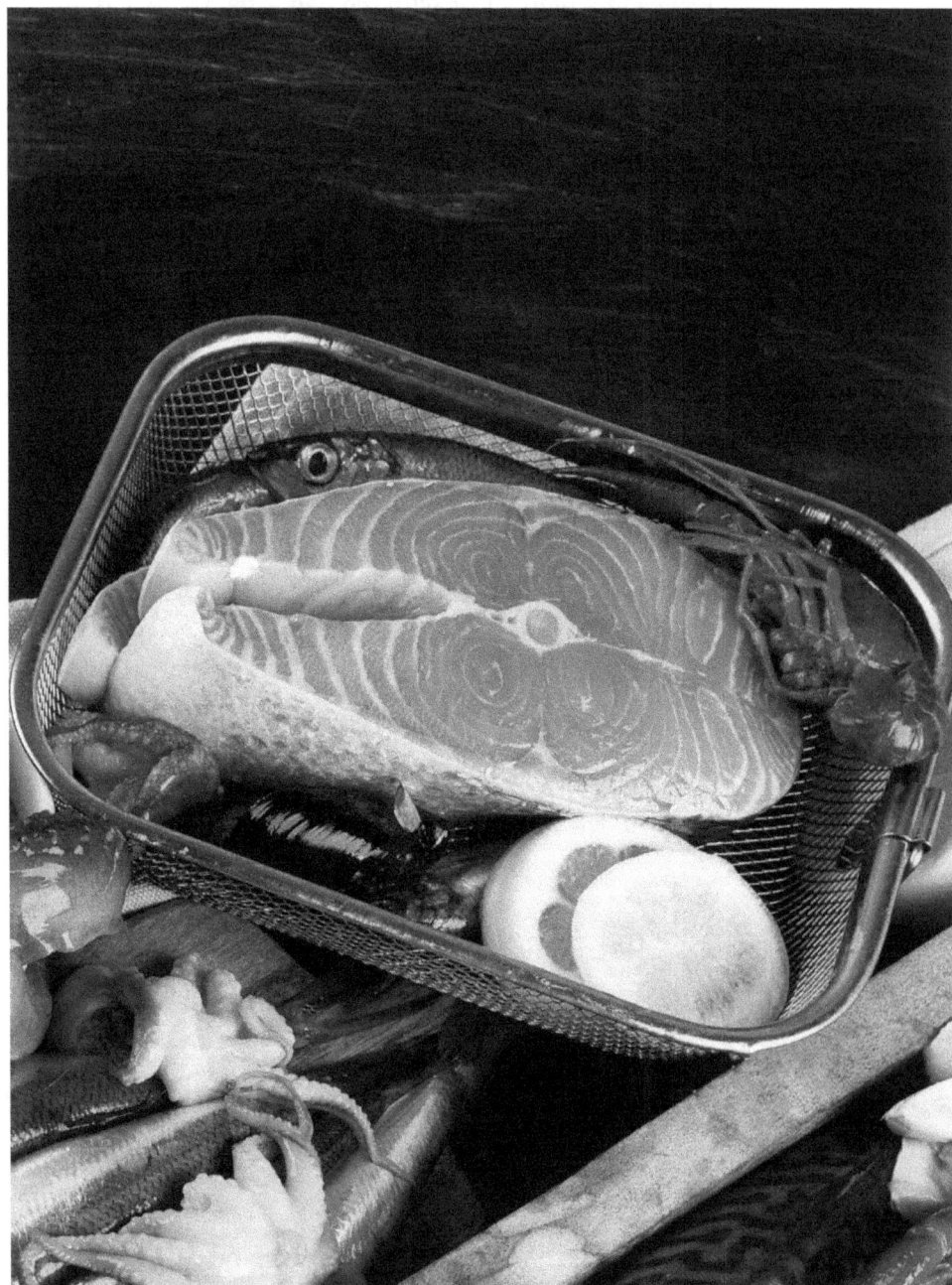

Poached Gennaro/Seabass with Red Peppers

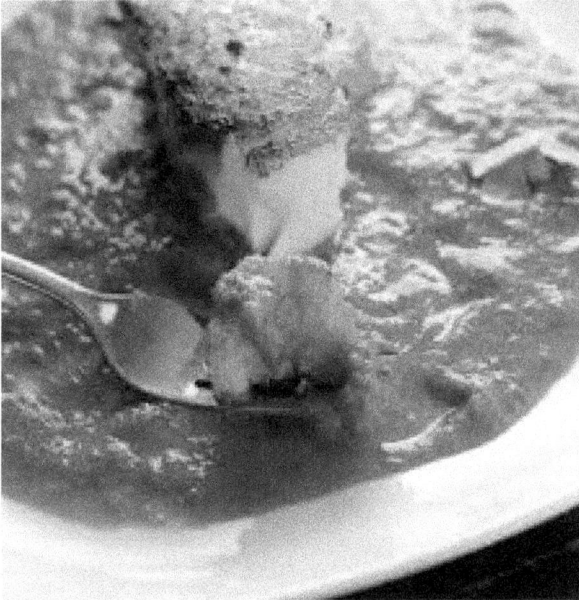

Preparation Time: 10 minutes

Cooking Time: 40 minutes

Serving: 1

INGREDIENTS:

- o 2 red peppers, trimmed
- o 11 oz Gennaro/seabass, trimmed
- o 1 teaspoon salt
- o ½ teaspoon ground black pepper
- o 2 tablespoons butter
- o 1 lemon

DIRECTIONS:

1) Remove the seeds from red peppers and cut them into wedges.
2) Then line the baking tray with parchment and arrange red peppers in a layer.

3) Rub Gennaro/seabass with ground black pepper and salt and place it on the peppers.
4) Then add butter.
5) Cut the lemon on the halves and squeeze the juice over the fish.
6) Bake the fish for 40 minutes at 350^0 F.

NUTRITION (Per Serving): Calories 148, Fat 10.3, Phosphorus: 36mg; Potassium: 194mg; Sodium: 31mg; Fiber 1.2, Carbs 7.3, Protein 8.5.

4-Ingredients Salmon Fillet

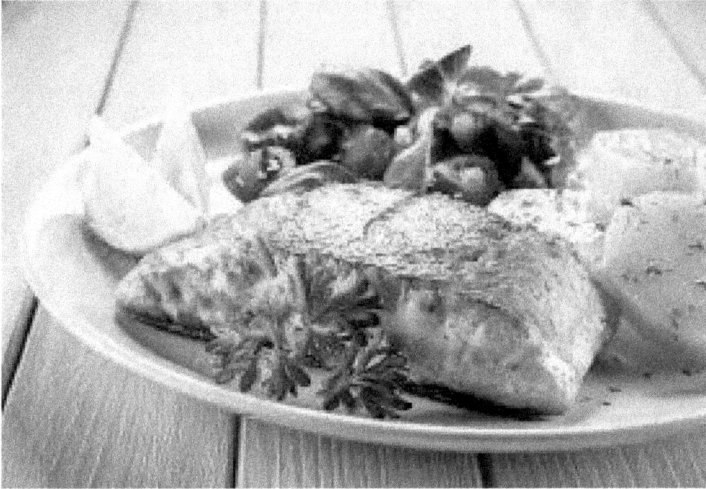

Preparation Time: 5 minutes

Cooking Time: 25 minutes

Serving: 1

INGREDIENTS:

- o 4 oz salmon fillet
- o ½ teaspoon salt
- o 1 teaspoon sesame oil
- o ½ teaspoon sage

DIRECTIONS:

1) Rub the fillet with salt and sage.
2) Place the fish in the tray and sprinkle it with sesame oil.
3) Cook the fish for 25 minutes at 365^0 F.
4) Flip the fish carefully onto another side after 12 minutes of cooking.

NUTRITION (Per Serving): Calories 191; Phosphorus: 30mg; Potassium: 74mg; Sodium: 30mg; Fat 11.6; Fiber 0.1; Carbs 0.2; Protein 22.

Spanish Cod in Sauce

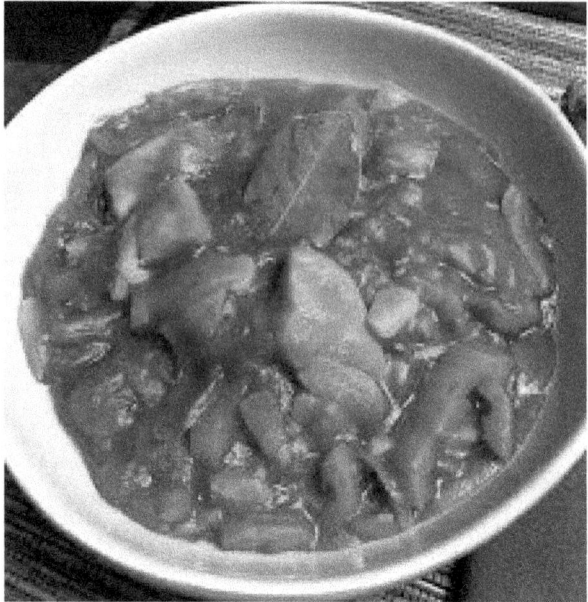

Preparation Time: 10 minutes

Cooking Time: 5.5 hours

Serving: 2

INGREDIENTS:

- o 1 teaspoon tomato paste
- o 1 teaspoon garlic, diced
- o 1 white onion, sliced
- o 1 jalapeno pepper, chopped
- o 1/3 cup chicken stock
- o 7 oz Spanish cod fillet
- o 1 teaspoon paprika
- o 1 teaspoon salt

DIRECTIONS:

1) Pour chicken stock in the saucepan.
2) Add tomato paste and mix up the liquid until homogenous.
3) Add garlic, onion, jalapeno pepper, paprika, and salt.
4) Bring the liquid to boil and then simmer it.
5) Chop the cod fillet and add it in the tomato liquid.
6) Close the lid and simmer the fish for 10 minutes over the low heat.
7) Serve the fish in the bowls with tomato sauce.

NUTRITION (Per Serving): Calories 113; Fat 1.2; Phosphorus: 54mg; Potassium: 24mg; Sodium: 22mg; Fiber 1.9; Carbs 7.2; Protein 18.9.

Oregano Grilled Calamari

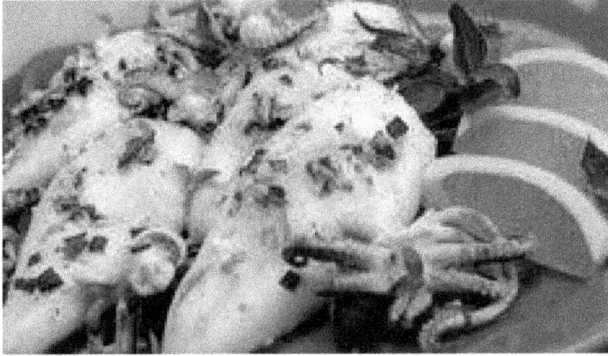

Preparation Time: 10 minutes

Cooking Time: 5 minutes

Serving: 1

INGREDIENTS:

- o 2 teaspoons garlic, minced
- o Pinch sea salt
- o 2 tablespoons olive oil
- o 2 tablespoons lemon juice
- o 1 tablespoon chopped fresh parsley
- o 1 tablespoon chopped fresh oregano
- o Pinch black pepper (ground)
- o ½ pound cleaned calamari
- o Lemon wedges

DIRECTIONS:

1) In a mixing bowl, add olive oil, lemon juice, parsley, oregano, garlic, salt, and pepper. Combine to mix well.
2) Add calamari and combine again. Refrigerate to marinate for 1 hour.
3) Preheat grill over medium heat setting; grease grates with some oil.

4) Grill calamari for 3 minutes, until evenly cooked. Turn halfway through.
5) Serve warm with some lemon wedges.

NUTRITION (Per Serving): Calories: 103; Fat: 6g; Phosphorus: 130mg; Potassium: 176mg; Sodium: 73mg; Carbohydrates: 2g; Protein: 4g.

Baked Shrimp Crabs

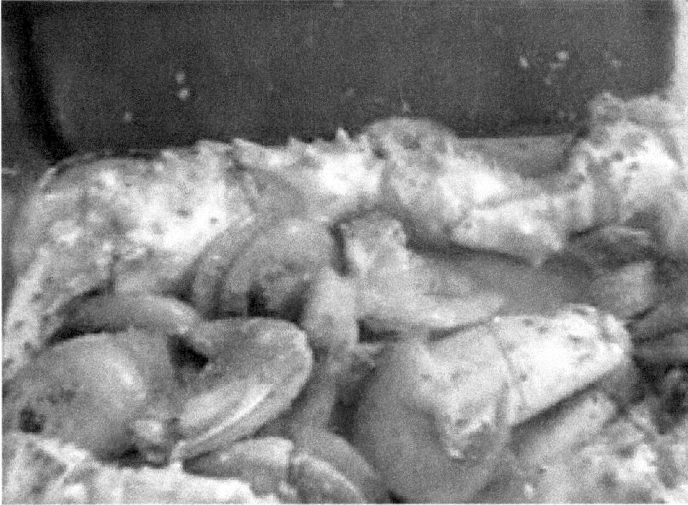

Preparation Time: 10 minutes

Cooking Time: 30 minutes

Serving: 1

INGREDIENTS:

- o 4 tablespoons green pepper, chopped
- o 2 tablespoons green onions, chopped
- o 1 cup celery, chopped
- o 1 cup crabmeat, cooked (boiled)
- o 1 cup shrimp, cooked (boiled)
- o ½ cup frozen green peas, thawed
- o ½ teaspoon black pepper
- o ½ cup mayonnaise
- o 1 cup breadcrumbs

DIRECTIONS:

1) Preheat the oven to 375ºF. Grease a casserole dish with some cooking spray.
2) In a mixing bowl, add all ingredients except breadcrumbs. Combine to mix well.
3) Add the mixture in a casserole dish and bake for 30 minutes until evenly brown.
4) Serve warm.

NUTRITION (Per Serving): Calories: 268; Fat: 7g; Phosphorus: 159mg; Potassium: 287mg; Sodium: 466mg; Carbohydrates: 21g; Protein: 17g.

Salmon Stuffed Pasta

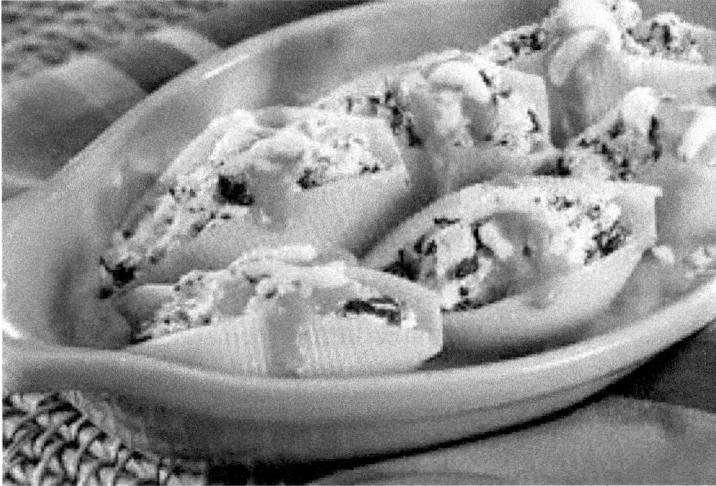

Preparation Time: 10 minutes

Cooking Time: 35 minutes

Serving: 1

INGREDIENTS:

- o   24 jumbo pasta shells, boiled
- o   1 cup coffee creamer

Filling:

- o   2 eggs, beaten
- o   2 cups creamed cottage cheese
- o   ¼ cup chopped onion
- o   1 red bell pepper, diced
- o   2 teaspoons dried parsley
- o   ½ teaspoon lemon peel
- o   1 can salmon, drained

Dill Sauce:

- o   1 ½ teaspoon butter
- o   1 ½ teaspoon flour

- ○ 1/8 teaspoon pepper
- ○ 1 tablespoon lemon juice
- ○ 1 ½ cup coffee creamer
- ○ 2 teaspoons dried dill weed

DIRECTIONS:

1) Beat the egg with the cream cheese and all the other filling ingredients in a bowl.
2) Divide the filling and fill in the pasta shells and place the shells in a 9x13 baking dish.
3) Pour the coffee creamer around the stuffed shells then cover with a foil.
4) Bake the shells for 30 minutes at 350^0 F.
5) Meanwhile, whisk all the ingredients for dill sauce in a saucepan.
6) Stir for 5 minutes, until it thickens.
7) Pour this sauce over the baked pasta shells.
8) Serve warm.

NUTRITION (Per Serving): Calories 268; Total Fat 4.8g; Saturated Fat 2g; Cholesterol 27mg; Sodium 86mg; Total Carbohydrate 42.6g; Dietary Fiber 2.1g; Sugars 2.4g; Protein 11.5g; Calcium 27mg; Phosphorous 314mg; Potassium 181mg.

Meat

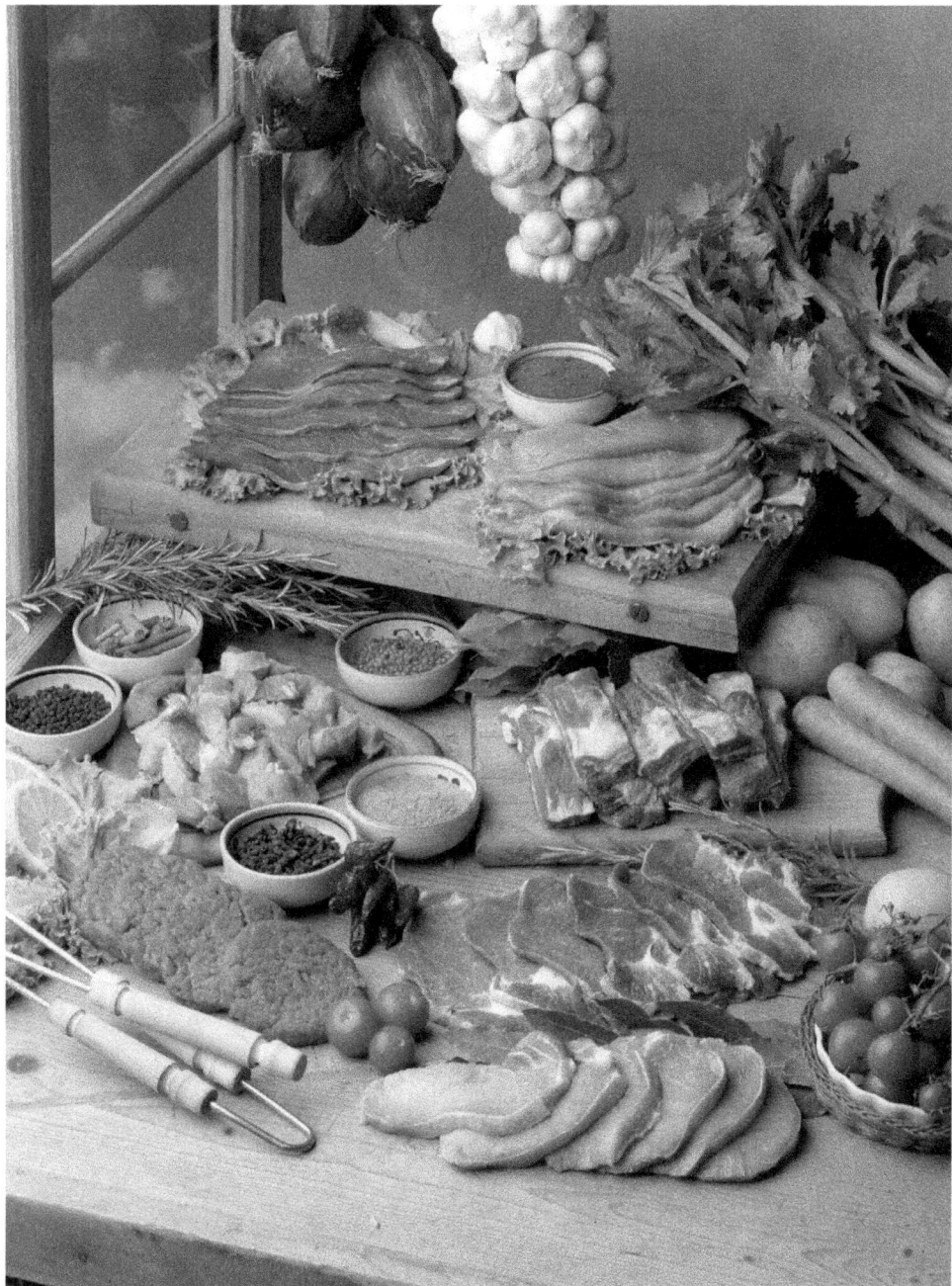

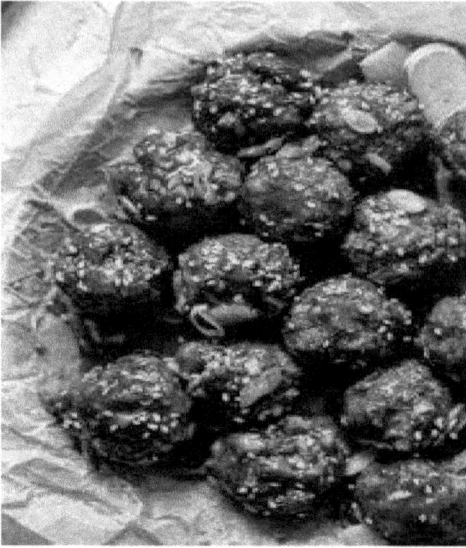

Baked Meatballs & Scallions

Preparation Time: 20 minutes

Cooking Time: 35 minutes

Serving: 1

INGREDIENTS:

For Meatballs:
- 1 lemongrass stalk, outer skin peeled and chopped
- 1 (1½-inch) piece fresh ginger, sliced
- 3 garlic cloves, chopped
- 1 cup fresh cilantro leaves, chopped roughly
- ½ cup fresh basil leaves, chopped roughly
- 2 tablespoons plus 1 teaspoon fish sauce
- 2 tablespoons water
- 2 tablespoons fresh lime juice
- ½ pound lean ground pork
- 1-pound lean ground lamb
- 1 carrot, peeled and grated
- 1 organic egg, beaten

For Scallions:

- 16 stalks scallions, trimmed
- 2 tablespoons coconut oil, melted
- Salt, to taste
- ½ cup water

DIRECTIONS:

1) Preheat the oven to 375^0 F. Grease a baking dish.
2) In a blender, add lemongrass, ginger, garlic, fresh herbs, fish sauce, water, and lime juice and pulse till chopped finely.
3) Transfer the mixture in a bowl, with the remaining ingredients and mix well.
4) Make about 1-inch balls from the mixture.
5) Arrange the balls into the prepared baking dish in a single layer.
6) In another rimmed baking dish, arrange scallion stalks in a single layer.
7) Drizzle with coconut oil and sprinkle with salt.
8) Pour water in the baking dish, then, with a foil paper, cover it tightly.
9) Bake the scallion for around a half-hour.
10) Bake the meatballs for approximately 30-35 minutes.
11) Serve the meatballs and scallion when done.

NUTRITION (Per Serving): Calories: 432; Fat: 13g; Phosphorus: 45mg; Potassium: 78mg; Sodium: 34mg; Carbohydrates: 25g; Fiber: 8g; Protein: 40g.

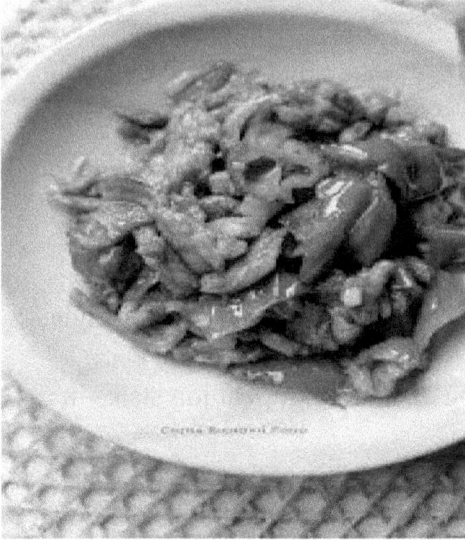

Pork with Bell Pepper

Preparation Time: 15 minutes

Cooking Time: 13 minutes

Serving: 1

INGREDIENTS:

- 1 tablespoon fresh ginger, chopped finely
- 4 garlic cloves, chopped finely
- 1 cup fresh cilantro, chopped and divided
- ¼ cup plus 1 tablespoon olive oil, divided
- 1-pound tender pork, trimmed, sliced thinly
- 2 onions, sliced thinly
- 1 green bell pepper, seeded and sliced thinly
- 1 tablespoon fresh lime juice

DIRECTIONS:

1) In a substantial bowl, mix ginger, garlic, ½ cup of cilantro, and ¼ cup of oil.
2) Add pork and coat with mixture generously.
3) Refrigerate to marinate, for a couple of hours.
4) Heat a big skillet on medium-high heat.
5) Add pork mixture and stir fry for approximately 4-5 minutes.
6) Transfer the pork right into a bowl.
7) In the same skillet, heat remaining oil on medium heat.
8) Add onion and sauté for approximately 3 minutes.
9) Stir in bell pepper and stir fry for about 3 minutes.

10) Stir in pork, lime juice, and remaining cilantro and cook for about 2 minutes.
11) Serve hot.

NUTRITION (Per Serving): Calories: 429; Fat: 19g; Phosphorus: 36mg; Potassium: 57mg; Sodium: 31mg; Carbohydrates: 26g; Fiber: 9g; Protein: 35g.

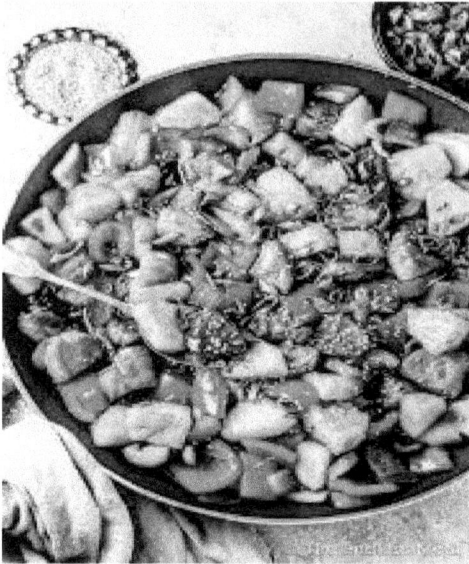

Pork with Pineapple

Preparation Time: 15 minutes

Cooking Time: 14 minutes

Serving: 1

INGREDIENTS:

o   2 tablespoons coconut oil
o   1½ pound pork tenderloin, trimmed and cut into bite-sized pieces
o   1 onion, chopped
o   2 minced garlic cloves
o   1 (1-inch) piece fresh ginger, minced
o   20-ounce pineapple, cut into chunks
o   1 large red bell pepper, seeded and chopped
o   ¼ cup fresh pineapple juice
o   ¼ cup coconut aminos
o   Salt and freshly ground black pepper, to taste

DIRECTIONS:

1) In a substantial skillet, melt coconut oil on high heat.
2) Add pork and stir fry approximately 4-5 minutes.
3) Transfer the pork into a bowl.
4) In the same skillet, heat remaining oil on medium heat.
5) Add onion, garlic, and ginger and sauté for around 2 minutes.
6) Stir in pineapple and bell pepper and stir fry for around 3 minutes.
7) Stir in pork, pineapple juice, and coconut aminos and cook for around 3-4 minutes.
8) Serve hot.

NUTRITION (Per Serving): Calories: 431; Fat: 10g; Phosphorus: 36mg; Potassium: 64mg; Sodium: 30mg; Carbohydrates: 22g; Fiber: 8g; Protein: 33g.

Spiced Pork

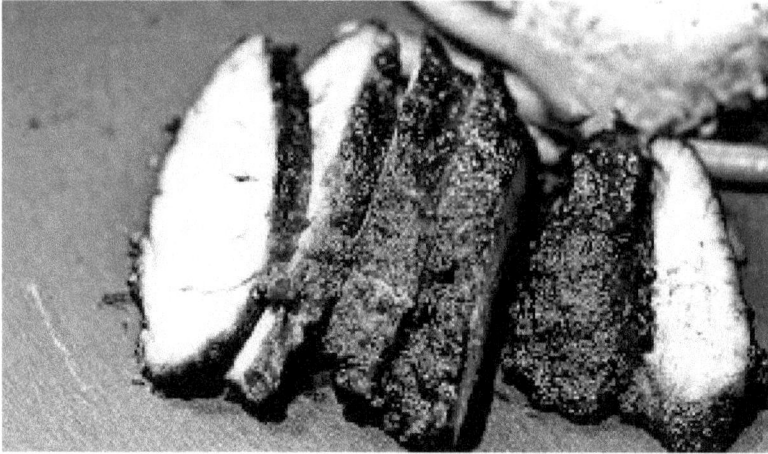

Preparation Time: 15 minutes

Cooking Time: 1 hour 52 minutes

Serving: 1

INGREDIENTS:

- o 1 (2-inch) piece fresh ginger, chopped
- o 5-10 garlic cloves, chopped
- o 1 teaspoon ground cumin
- o ½ teaspoon ground turmeric
- o 1 tablespoon hot paprika
- o 1 tablespoon red pepper flakes
- o Salt, to taste
- o 2 tablespoons cider vinegar
- o 2-pounds pork shoulder, trimmed and cubed into 1½-inch size
- o 2 cups domestic hot water, divided
- o 1 (1-inch wide) ball tamarind pulp
- o ¼ cup olive oil
- o 1 teaspoon black mustard seeds, crushed
- o 4 green cardamoms
- o 5 whole cloves
- o 1 (3-inch) cinnamon stick

- ○ 1 cup onion, chopped finely
- ○ 1 large red bell pepper, seeded and chopped

DIRECTIONS:

1) In a food processor, add ginger, garlic, cumin, turmeric, paprika, red pepper flakes, salt, and cider vinegar, and pulse till smooth.
2) Transfer the mixture into a large bowl.
3) Add pork and coat it with the mixture generously.
4) Keep aside, covered for around an hour at room temperature.
5) In a bowl, add 1 cup of warm water and tamarind and keep aside till water cools.
6) With the hands, crush the tamarind to extract the pulp.
7) Add remaining cup of hot water and mix till well combined.
8) Through a fine sieve, strain the tamarind juice in a bowl.
9) In a skillet, heat oil on medium-high heat.
10) Add mustard seeds, green cardamoms, cloves, and cinnamon stick and sauté for about 4 minutes.
11) Add onion and sauté for around 5 minutes.
12) Add pork and stir fry for approximately 6 minutes.
13) Stir in tamarind juice and let it come to a boil.
14) Reduce the heat to medium-low and simmer for 1½ hours.
15) Stir in bell pepper and cook for about 7 minutes.

NUTRITION (Per Serving): Calories: 435; Fat: 16g; Phosphorus: 28mg; Potassium: 64mg; Sodium: 19mg; Carbohydrates: 27g; Fiber: 3g; Protein: 39g.

Pork Chili

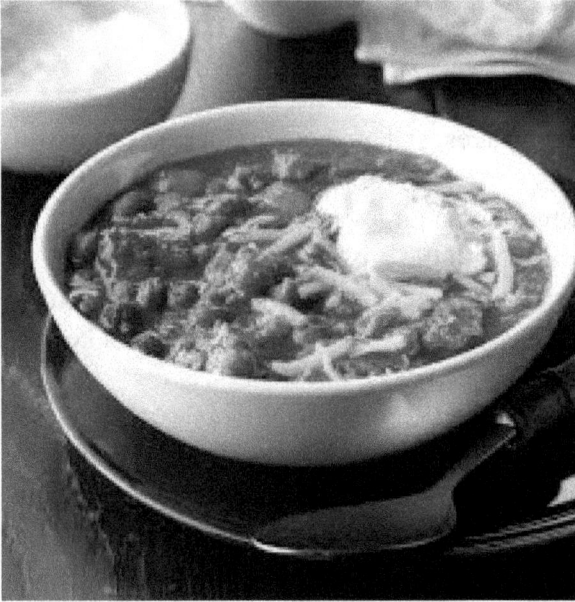

Preparation Time: 15 minutes

Cooking Time: 1 hour

Serving: 1

INGREDIENTS:

- o 2 tablespoons extra-virgin organic olive oil
- o 2-pound ground pork
- o 1 medium red bell pepper, seeded and chopped
- o 1 medium onion, chopped
- o 5 garlic cloves, chopped finely
- o 1 (2-inch) part of hot pepper, minced
- o 1 tablespoon ground cumin
- o 1 teaspoon ground turmeric
- o 3 tablespoon chili powder
- o ½ teaspoon chipotle chili powder
- o Salt and freshly ground black pepper, to taste
- o 1 cup chicken broth

- o   1 (28-ounce) can fire-roasted crushed tomatoes
- o   2 medium Bok choy heads, sliced
- o   1 avocado, peeled, pitted, and chopped

DIRECTIONS:

1) In a sizable pan, heat oil on medium heat.
2) Add pork and stir fry for about 5 minutes.
3) Add bell pepper, onion, garlic, hot pepper, and spices and stir fry for approximately 5 minutes.
4) Add broth and tomatoes and convey with a boil.
5) Stir in Bok choy and cook, covered for approximately twenty minutes.
6) Uncover and cook for approximately 20 minutes to half an hour.
7) Serve hot while using a topping of avocado.

NUTRITION (Per Serving): Calories: 402; Fat: 9g; Phosphorus: 20mg; Potassium: 156mg; Sodium: 34mg; Carbohydrates: 18g; Fiber: 6g; Protein: 32g.

Ground Pork with Water Chestnuts

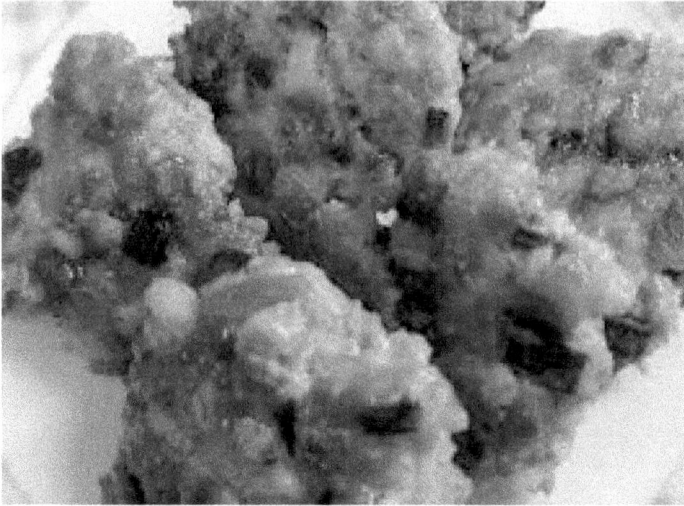

Preparation Time: 15 minutes

Cooking Time: 12 minutes

Serving: 1

INGREDIENTS:

- 1 tablespoon plus 1 teaspoon coconut oil
- 1 tablespoon fresh ginger, minced
- 1 bunch scallion (white and green parts separated), chopped
- 1-pound lean ground pork
- Salt, to taste
- 1 tablespoon 5-spice powder
- 1 (18-ounce) can water chestnuts, drained and chopped
- 1 tablespoon organic honey
- 2 tablespoons fresh lime juice

DIRECTIONS:

1) In a big heavy-bottomed skillet, heat oil on high heat.
2) Add ginger and scallion whites and sauté for approximately ½-1½ minutes.

3) Add pork and cook for approximately 4-5 minutes.
4) Drain the extra fat from the skillet.
5) Add salt and 5-spice powder and cook for approximately 2-3 minutes.
6) Add scallion greens and remaining ingredients and cook, stirring continuously for about 1-2 minutes.

NUTRITION (Per Serving): Calories: 520; Fat: 30g; Phosphorus: 20mg; Potassium: 120mg; Sodium: 9mg; Carbohydrates: 37g; Fiber: 4g; Protein: 25g.

Hearty Meatloaf

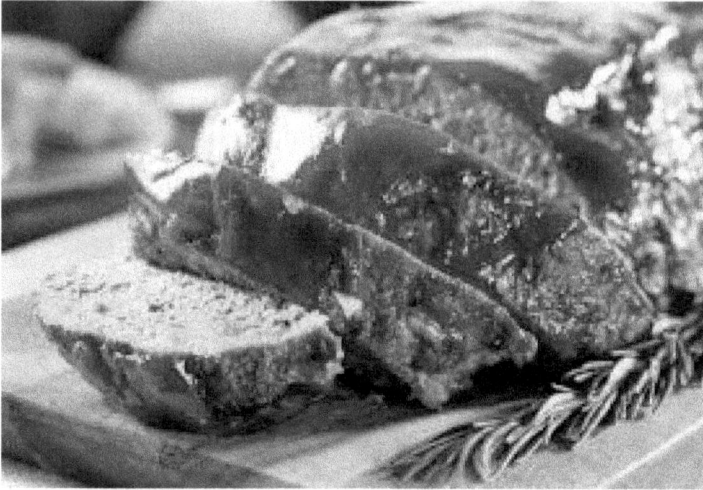

Preparation Time: 10 minutes

Cooking Time: 45-50 minutes

Serving: 1

INGREDIENTS:

- o   1 large egg
- o   2 tablespoons chopped fresh basil
- o   1 teaspoon chopped fresh thyme
- o   1 teaspoon chopped fresh parsley
- o   ¼ teaspoon black pepper (ground)
- o   1 pound 95% lean ground beef
- o   ½ cup breadcrumbs
- o   ½ cup chopped sweet onion
- o   1 teaspoon white vinegar
- o   ¼ teaspoon garlic powder
- o   1 tablespoon brown sugar

DIRECTIONS:

1) Preheat an oven to 350ºF. Grease a loaf pan (9X5-inch) with some cooking spray.
2) In a mixing bowl, add beef, breadcrumbs, onion, egg, basil, thyme, parsley, and black pepper. Combine to mix.
3) Add the mixture in the pan.
4) Take another mixing bowl; add brown sugar, vinegar, and garlic powder. Combine to mix well.
5) Add brown sugar mixture over the meat mixture.
6) Bake for about 50 minutes until golden brown.
7) Serve warm.

NUTRITION (Per Serving): Calories: 118; Fat: 3g; Phosphorus: 127mg; Potassium: 203mg; Sodium: 106mg; Carbohydrates: 8g; Protein: 12g.

Chicken with Mushrooms

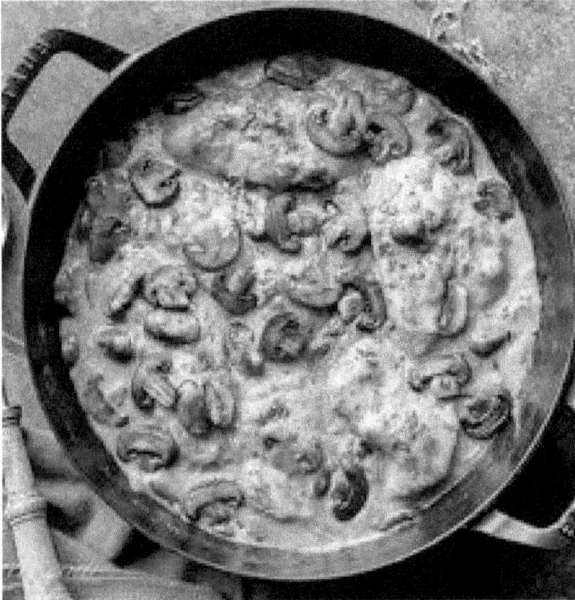

Preparation Time: 15 minutes

Cooking Time: 45 minutes

Serving: 2

INGREDIENTS:

- o 2 tablespoon light sour cream
- o ¼ cup all-purpose flour
- o 1 cup no salt added chicken broth
- o 1 tablespoon Dijon mustard
- o ¼ teaspoon dried thyme
- o 4 chicken breasts
- o 1½ cups mushrooms, quartered
- o 1 tablespoon nonhydrogenated margarine
- o Fresh ground pepper and chopped fresh parsley, to taste
- o 3 chopped green onions

DIRECTIONS:

1) Mix 2 tablespoon of chicken broth, mustard, sour cream, and 2 teaspoon flour. Set aside.
2) Sprinkle chicken with pepper and thyme. Dredge in flour.
3) Melt margarine on medium-low heat in a large non-stick pan. Cook chicken for 15-20 minutes per side. Remove from heat and keep warm.
4) Add mushrooms to another pan. Increase the heat and boil for 3 minutes.
5) Add sour cream mixture and green onions and cook until thickened.
6) Pour over chicken. Garnish with parsley and pepper.

NUTRIENTS per Serving: Protein-25.4g; Phosphorus: 29mg; Potassium: 142mg; Sodium: 17mg; Carbohydrates-5g; Fat - 4g; Calories – 161.

Vegetable

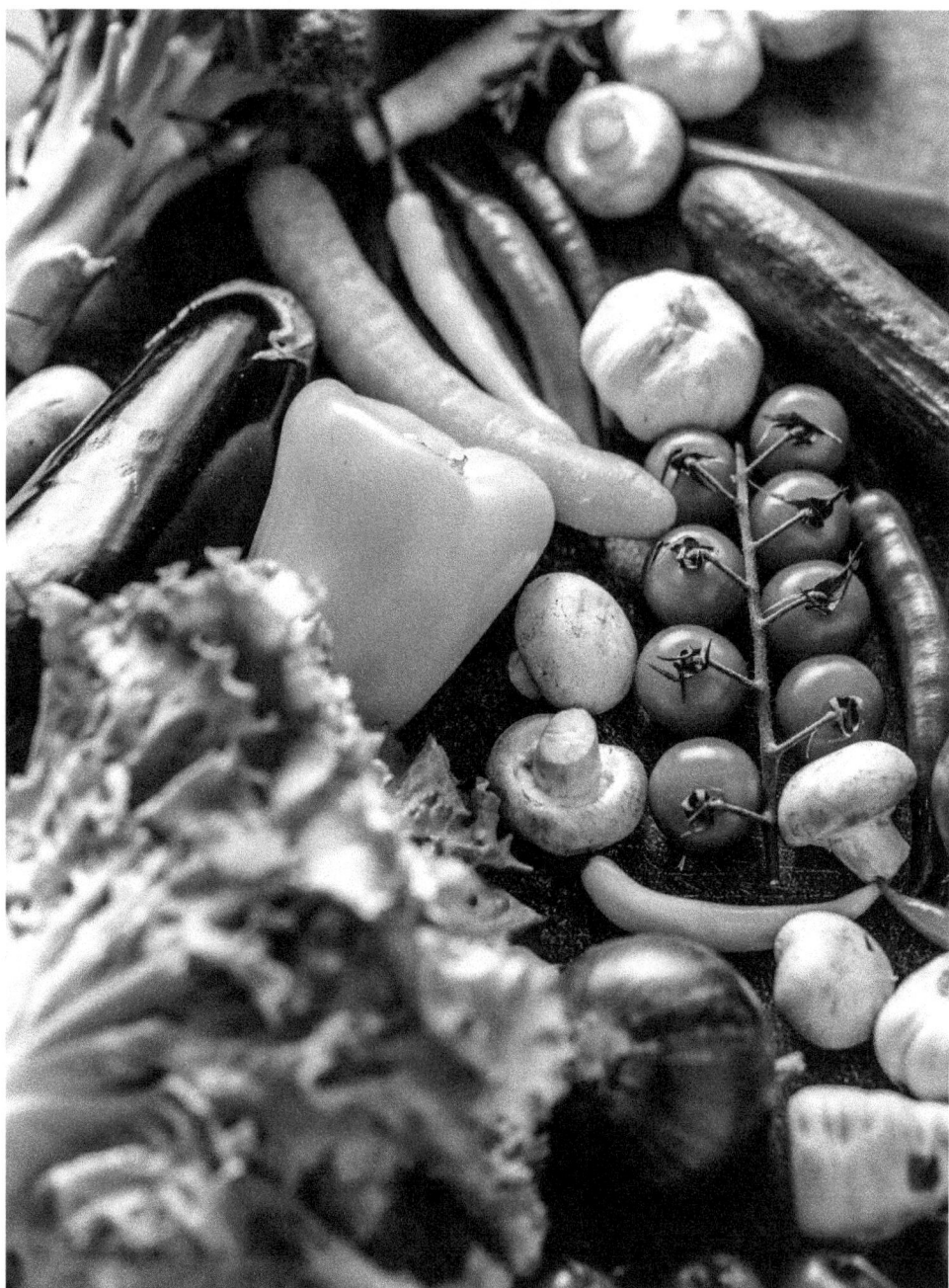

Cauliflower Fritters

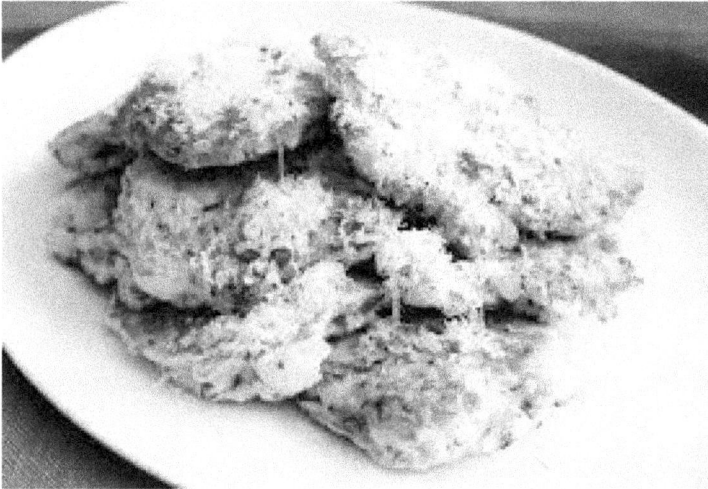

Preparation Time: 10 minutes

Cooking Time: 15 minutes

Serving: 1

INGREDIENTS:

- o 1 large cauliflower head, cut into florets
- o 2 eggs, beaten
- o ½ teaspoon turmeric
- o ½ teaspoon salt
- o ¼ teaspoon black pepper
- o 1 tablespoon coconut oil

DIRECTIONS:

1) Place the cauliflower florets in a pot with water and bring to a boil. Cook until tender, until around 5 minutes of boiling. Drain well.
2) Place the cauliflower, eggs, turmeric, salt, and pepper into the food processor.
3) Pulse until the mixture becomes coarse.

4) Transfer into a bowl. Using your hands, form six small flattened balls and place in the fridge for at least 1 hour, until the mixture hardens.
5) Heat the oil in a nonstick pan and fry the cauliflower patties for 3 minutes on each side.
6) Serve and enjoy.

NUTRITION (Per Serving): Calories 53; Total Fat 6g; Saturated Fat 2g; Total Carbs 2g; Net Carbs 1g; Protein 3g; Sugar: 1g; Fiber 1g; Sodium 228mg; Potassium 159mg.

Stir-Fried Squash

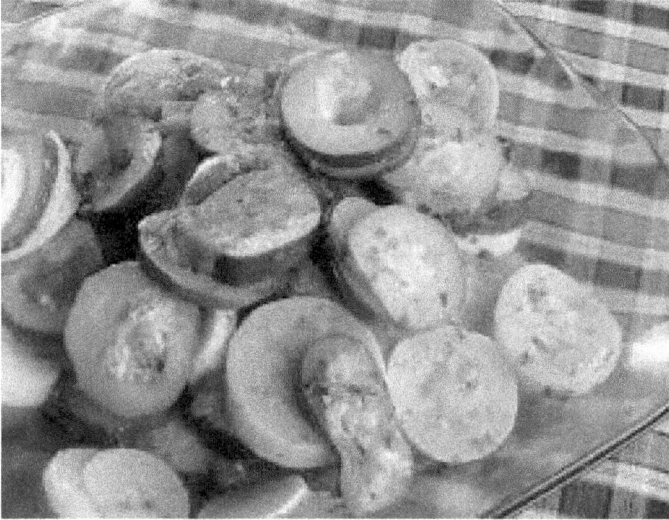

Preparation Time: 10 minutes

Cooking Time: 10 minutes

Serving: 1

INGREDIENTS:

- o 1 tablespoon olive oil
- o 3 cloves of garlic, minced
- o 1 butternut squash, seeded and sliced
- o 1 tablespoon coconut aminos
- o 1 tablespoon lemon juice
- o 1 tablespoon water
- o Salt and pepper to taste

DIRECTIONS:

1) Heat oil over medium flame and sauté the garlic until fragrant.
2) Stir in the squash for another 3 minutes before adding the rest of the ingredients.

3) Close the lid and allow to simmer for 5 more minutes or until the squash is soft.
4) Serve and enjoy.

NUTRITION (Per Serving): Calories 83; Total Fat 3g; Saturated Fat 0.5g; Total Carbs 14g; Net Carbs 12g; Protein 2g; Sugar: 1g; Fiber 2g; Sodium 8mg; Potassium 211mg.

Cauliflower Hash Brown

Preparation Time: 10 minutes

Cooking Time: 20 minutes

Serving: 1

INGREDIENTS:

- 4 eggs, beaten
- ½ cup coconut milk
- ½ teaspoon dry mustard
- Salt and pepper to taste
- 1 large head cauliflower, shredded

DIRECTIONS:

1) Place all ingredients in a mixing bowl and mix until well combined.
2) Place a nonstick frypan and heat over medium flame.
3) Add a large dollop of cauliflower mixture in the skillet.
4) Fry one side for 3 minutes, flip and cook the other side for a minute, like a pancake. Repeat process to remaining ingredients.
5) Serve and enjoy.

NUTRITION (Per Serving): Calories 102; Total Fat 8g; Saturated Fat 1g; Total Carbs 4g; Net Carbs 3g; Protein 5g; Sugar: 2g; Fiber 1g; Sodium 63mg; Potassium 251mg

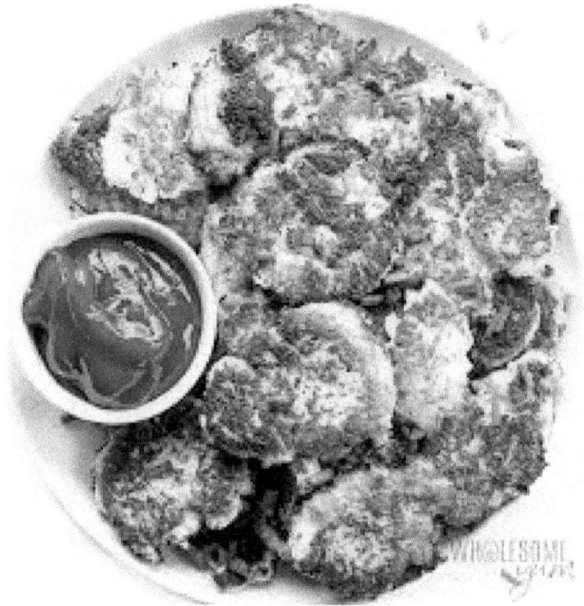

Sweet Potato Puree

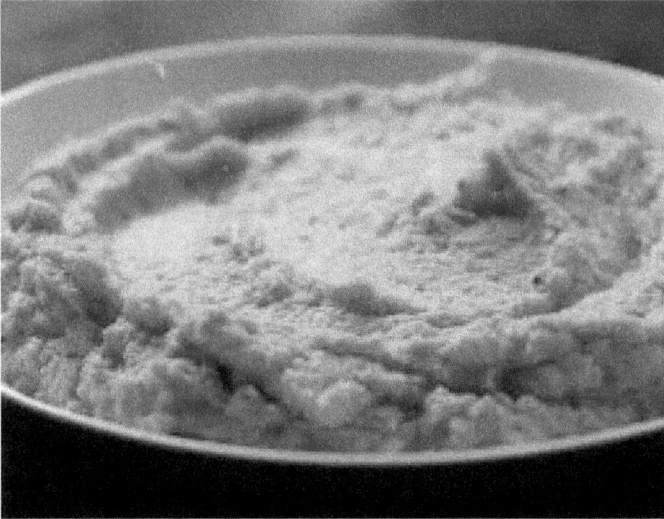

Preparation Time: 10 minutes

Cooking Time: 15 minutes

Serving: 1

INGREDIENTS:

- o 2 pounds sweet potatoes; peeled
- o 1½ cups water
- o 5 Medjool dates; pitted and chopped

DIRECTIONS:

1) Place water and potatoes in a pot.
2) Close the lid and allow to boil for 15 minutes until the potatoes are soft.
3) Drain the potatoes and place them in a food processor together with the dates.
4) Pulse until smooth.
5) Serve and enjoy.

NUTRITION (Per Serving): Calories 172; Total Fat 0.2g; Saturated Fat 0g; Total Carbs 41g; Net Carbs 36g; Protein 3g; Sugar: 14g; Fiber 5g; Sodium 10mg; Potassium 776mg

Curried Okra

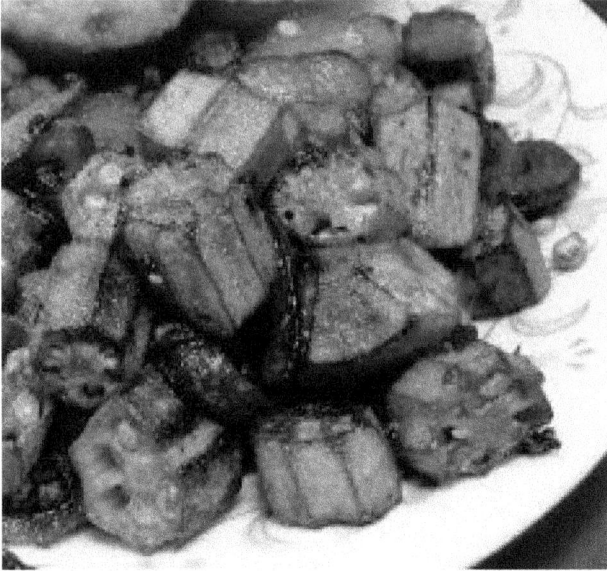

Preparation Time: 10 minutes

Cooking Time: 12 minutes

Serving: 1

INGREDIENTS:

- o   1 lb. small to medium okra pods; trimmed
- o   ¼ teaspoon curry powder
- o   ½ teaspoon kosher salt
- o   1 teaspoon finely chopped serrano chile
- o   1 teaspoon ground coriander
- o   1 tablespoon canola oil
- o   ¾ teaspoon brown mustard seeds

DIRECTIONS:

1) On medium-high fire; place a large and heavy skillet and cook mustard seeds until fragrant; around 30 seconds.
2) Add canola oil. Add okra; curry powder; salt; chile; and coriander. Sauté for a minute while stirring every once in a while.
3) Cover and cook on low flame for at least 8 minutes. Stir occasionally.
4) Uncover; increase the fire to medium-high and cook until okra is lightly browned; around 2 minutes more.
5) Serve and enjoy.

NUTRITION (Per Serving): Calories 78; Total Fat 6g; Saturated Fat 0.7g; Total Carbs 6g; Net Carbs 3g; Protein 2g; Sugar: 3g; Fiber 3g; Sodium 553mg; Potassium 187mg

Classic asparagus

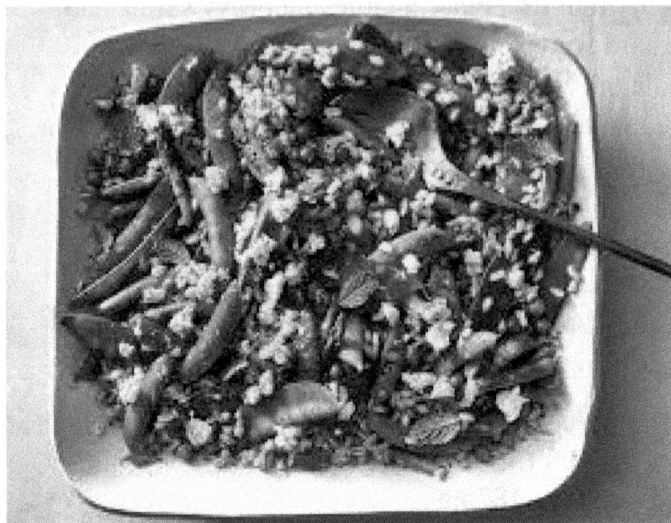

Preparation Time: 10 minutes

Cooking Time: 4-6 minutes

Serving: 1

INGREDIENTS:

- o 2 kg of white asparagus
- o 12 pieces of medium potatoes
- o 4 eggs
- o 1 first-class salt
- o 1 premium sugar
- o 1 tablespoon butter

For the Sauce

- o 200 g butter
- o 2 egg yolks
- o 4 tablespoons white wine
- o 1 tablespoon lemon juice
- o 1 first-class salt

o 1 premium white pepper

DIRECTIONS:

1) Cook the peeled asparagus in plenty of hot water (seasoned with salt, sugar, and butter) for 15 - 20 minutes.
2) Peel the potatoes and cook as usual and cool with the air freezer. The eggs are cooked hard.
3) <u>For the sauce:</u> Dissolve the butter in a hot freezer and allow cooling slightly.
4) Grease the egg yolks with lemon juice and white wine in a warm water bath until the mass is thick.
5) Then the cooled and melted butter is slowed down slowly. Now the sauce is seasoned with salt and pepper.

NUTRITION (Per Serving): Calories 20 % daily value; Total fat 0.1 g 0%; Saturated fat 0 g 0%; Total carbohydrate 3.9 g 1%; Phosphorus: 89mg; Potassium: 156mg; Sodium: 41mg; Dietary fiber 2.1 g 8%; Sugar 1.9 g; Protein 2.2 g 4%.

Soup cream from palm heart

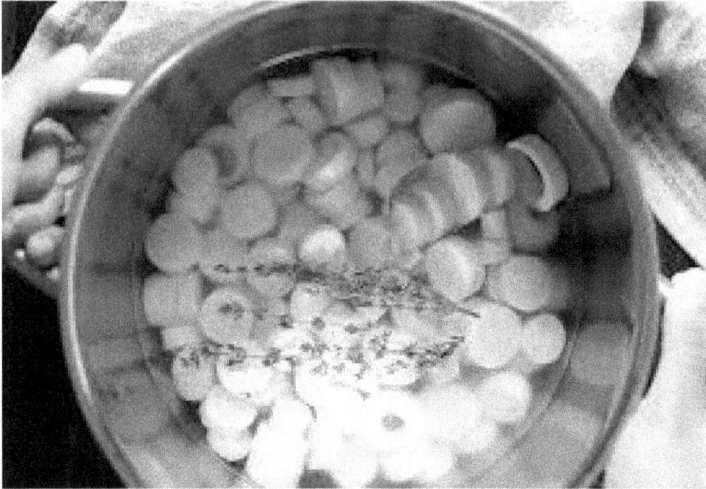

Preparation Time: 10 minutes

Cooking Time: 4-6 minutes

Serving: 1

INGREDIENTS:

- o 250g Pupunha palm
- o 3 cups of chicken broth tea
- o 1 cup skimmed milk
- o 1 tablespoon light margarine
- o 1 grated onion
- o 1 garlic kernel; chopped
- o Two tablespoons of wheat flour
- o Small salt

DIRECTIONS:

1) Onions and garlic must be sweetened in light margarine. Then add the Pupunha palm heart and pick up a little more to absorb the spice flavor.
2) It takes 2 to 3 minutes.

3) Dissolve wheat flour in chicken broth tea. It takes approximately 10 mins.
4) When it is lukewarm, apply the milk by adding skimmed milk. Go back to the fire for another 5 or 6 minutes. It's time to taste the salt. Serve immediately.

NUTRITION (Per Serving): Calories per **Serving:** about 62 calories, Phosphorus: 27mg; Potassium: 124mg; Sodium: 27mg;

Dessert

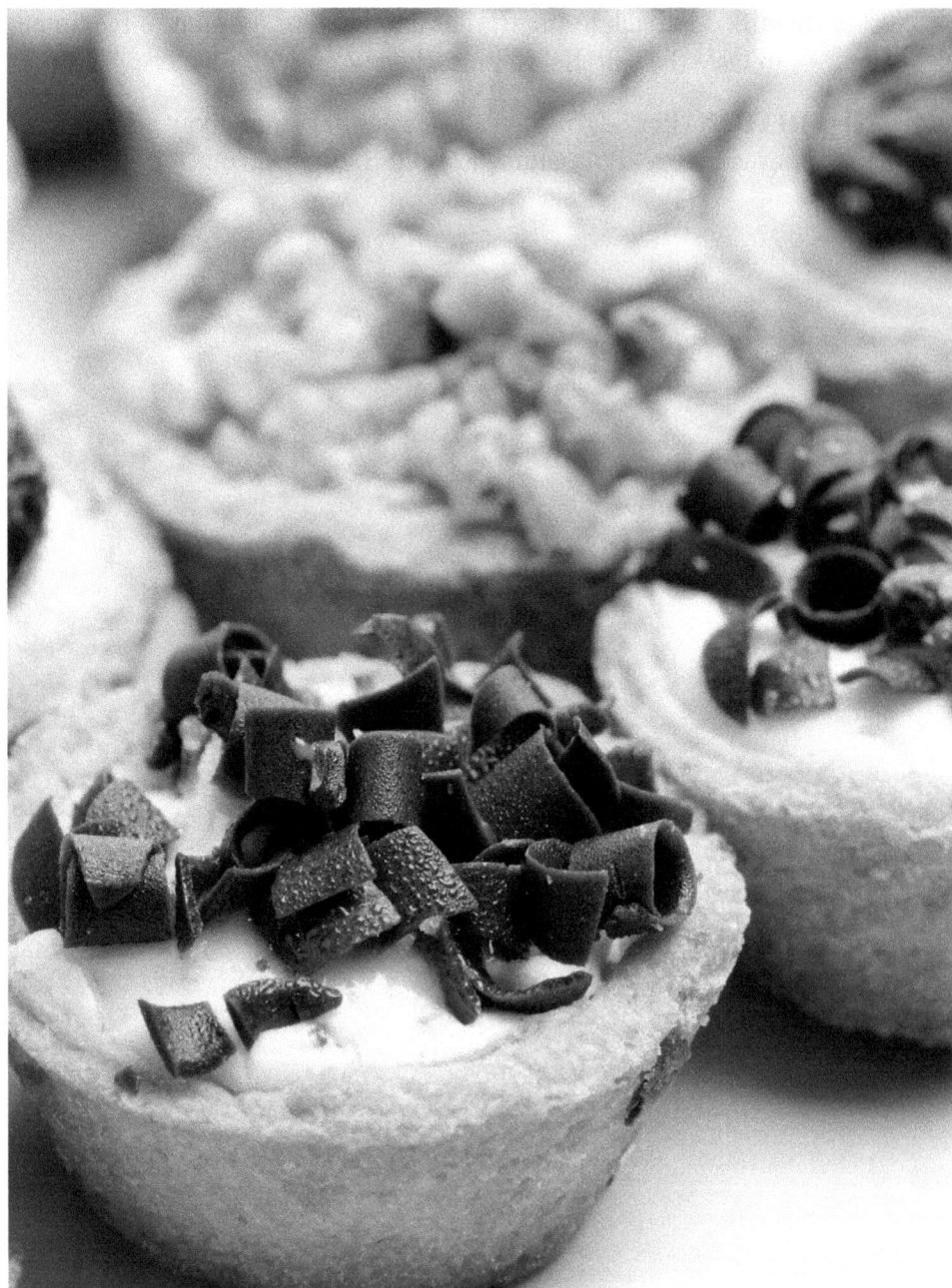

Grilled Pineapple

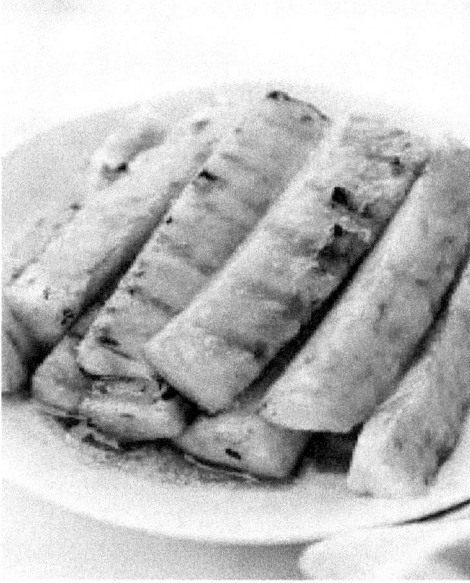

Preparation Time: 7 minutes

Cooking Time: 5 minutes

Serving: 1

INGREDIENTS:

- o   10 oz fresh pineapple
- o   ½ teaspoon ground ginger
- o   1 tablespoon almond butter, softened

DIRECTIONS:

1) Slice the pineapple into the serving pieces and brush with almond butter.
2) After this, sprinkle every pineapple piece with ground ginger.
3) Preheat the grill to 400^0 F.
4) Grill the pineapple for 2 minutes from each side.

5) The cooked fruit should have a light brown surface on both the sides.

NUTRITION (Per Serving): calories 61; fat 2.4; fiber 1.4; Phosphorus: 30mg; Potassium: 104mg; Sodium: 19mg; carbs 10.2; protein 1.3.

Coconut-Mint Bars

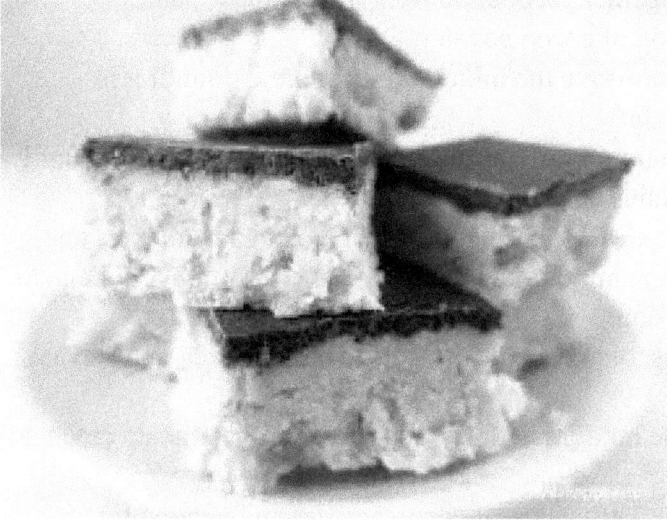

Preparation Time: 35 minutes

Cooking Time: 1 minute

Serving: 1

INGREDIENTS:

- o 3 tablespoons coconut butter
- o ½ cup coconut flakes
- o 1 egg, beaten
- o 1 tablespoon cocoa powder
- o 3 oz graham crackers, crushed
- o 2 tablespoons Erythritol
- o 3 tablespoons butter
- o 1 teaspoon mint extract
- o 1 teaspoon stevia powder
- o 1 teaspoon of cocoa powder
- o 1 tablespoon almond butter, melted

DIRECTIONS:

1) Churn together coconut butter, coconut flakes, and 1 tablespoon of cocoa powder.
2) Then microwave the mixture for 1 minute or until it is melted.
3) Chill the liquid for 1 minute and fast add egg. Whisk it until homogenous and smooth.
4) Add and stir the liquid in the crushed graham crackers and transfer the mixture to the mold. Flatten it well with the help of the spoon.
5) After this, blend Erythritol, butter, mint extract, and stevia powder.
6) When the mixture is fluffy; place it over the graham crackers layer.
7) Then mix 1 teaspoon of cocoa powder and almond butter.
8) Sprinkle the cocoa liquid on the cooked mixture and flatten it.
9) Refrigerate the dessert for 30 minutes.
10) Then cut it into the bars.

NUTRITION (Per Serving): Calories 213; Fat 16.3; Phosphorus: 20mg; Potassium: 154mg; Sodium: 10mg; Fiber 2.9; Carbs 20; Protein 3.5.

Lemon Mousse

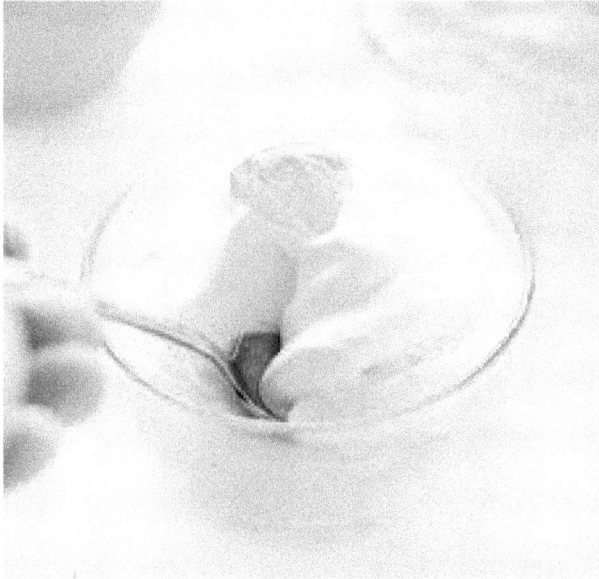

Preparation Time: 10 minutes + chill time

Cooking Time: 10 minutes

Serving: 1

INGREDIENTS:

- o 1 cup coconut cream
- o 8 ounces cream cheese; soft
- o ¼ cup fresh lemon juice
- o 3 pinches salt
- o 1 teaspoon lemon liquid stevia

DIRECTIONS:

1) Preheat your oven to 350°F
2) Grease a ramekin with butter.
3) Beat the cream, cream cheese, fresh lemon juice, salt, and lemon liquid stevia in a mixer.
4) Pour batter into the ramekin.

5) Bake for 10 minutes, then transfer the mousse to a serving glass.
6) Let it chill for 2 hours and serve.
7) Enjoy!

NUTRITION (Per Serving): Calories: 395; Fat: 31g; Phosphorus: 18mg; Potassium: 108mg; Sodium: 18mg; Carbohydrates: 3g; Protein: 5g.

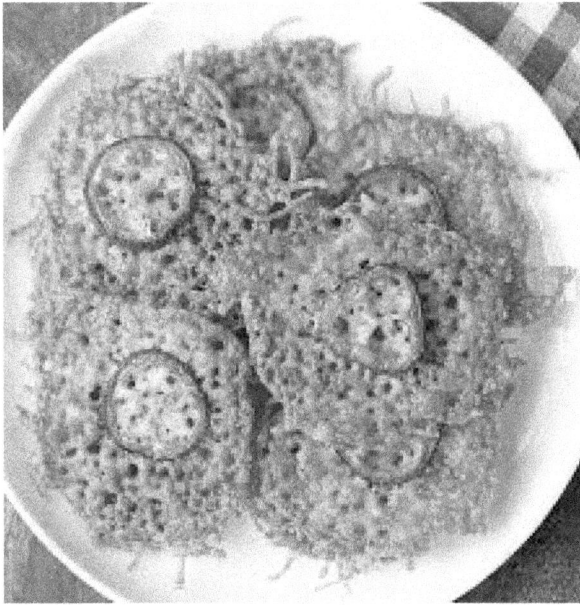

Jalapeno Crisp

Preparation Time: 10 minutes

Cooking Time: 1 hour 15 minutes

Serving: 2

INGREDIENTS:

- o 1 cup sesame seeds
- o 1 cup sunflower seeds
- o 1 cup flaxseeds
- o ½ cup hulled hemp seeds
- o 3 tablespoons Psyllium husk
- o 1 teaspoon salt
- o 1 teaspoon baking powder
- o 2 cups of water

DIRECTIONS:

1) Preheat your oven to 350°F
2) Take your blender and add seeds, baking powder, salt, and Psyllium husk.
3) Blend well until a sand-like texture appears.
4) Stir in water and mix until a batter form.
5) Allow the batter to rest for 10 minutes until a dough-like thick mixture forms.
6) Pour the dough onto a cookie sheet lined with parchment paper.

7) Spread it evenly, making sure that it has a thickness of ¼ inch all around.
8) Bake for 75 minutes in the oven.
9) Remove and cut it into pieces.
10) Allow them to cool for 30 minutes and enjoy!

NUTRITION (Per Serving): Calories: 156; Fat: 13g; Phosphorus: 10mg; Potassium: 70mg; Sodium: 17mg; Carbohydrates: 2g; Protein: 5g.

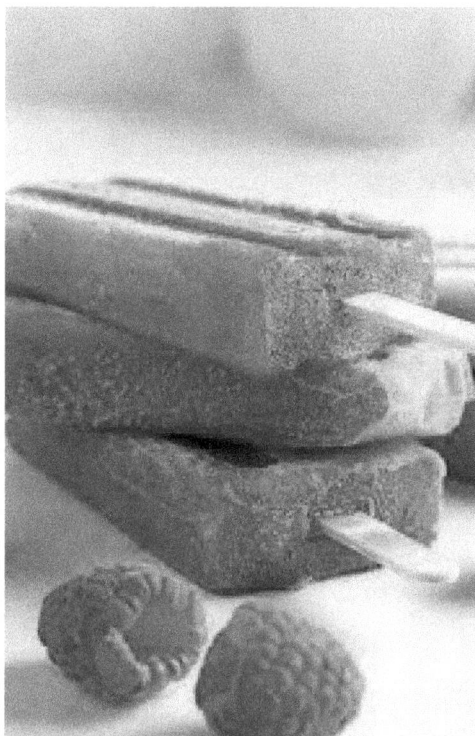

Raspberry Popsicle

Preparation Time: 2 hours

Cooking Time: 15 minutes

Serving: 1

INGREDIENTS:

- 1 ½ cups raspberries
- 2 cups of water

DIRECTIONS:

1) Take a pan and fill it up with water.
2) Add raspberries.
3) Place it over medium heat and bring to water to a boil.
4) Reduce the heat and simmer for 15 minutes.
5) Remove from the heat and pour the mix into popsicle molds.
6) Add a popsicle stick and let it chill for 2 hours.
7) Serve and enjoy!

NUTRITION (Per Serving): Calories: 58; Fat: 0.4g; Phosphorus: 30mg; Potassium: 114mg; Sodium: 21mg; Carbohydrates: 0g; Protein: 1.4g.

Easy Fudge

Preparation Time: 15 minutes + cooling time

Cooking Time: 5 minutes

Serving: 2

INGREDIENTS:

- o 1 ¾ cups of coconut butter
- o 1 cup pumpkin puree
- o 1 teaspoon ground cinnamon
- o ¼ teaspoon ground nutmeg
- o 1 tablespoon coconut oil

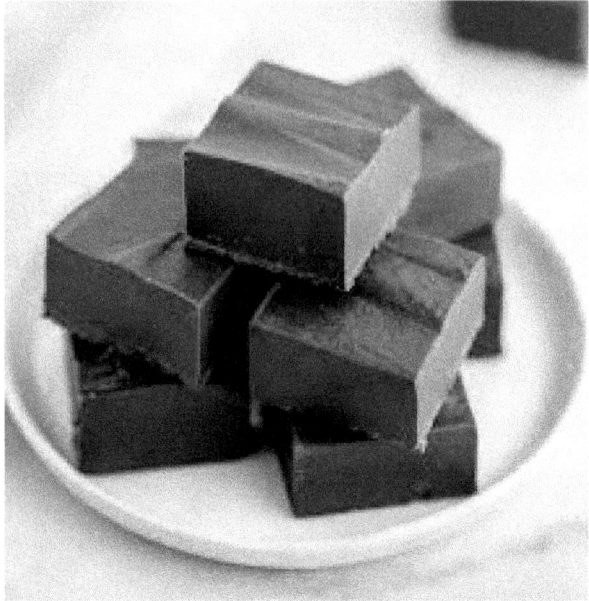

DIRECTIONS:

1) Take an 8x8 inch square baking pan and line it with aluminum foil.
2) Take a spoon and scoop out the coconut butter into a heated pan and allow the butter to melt.
3) Keep stirring well and remove from the heat once fully melted.
4) Add spices and pumpkin and keep straining until you have a grain-like texture.
5) Add coconut oil and keep stirring to incorporate everything.
6) Scoop the mixture into your baking pan and evenly distribute it
7) Place wax paper on top of the mixture and press gently to straighten the top
8) Remove the paper and discard it.

9) Allow the mixture to chill for 1-2 hours.
10) Once chilled, take it out and slice it up into pieces
11) Enjoy!

NUTRITION (Per Serving): Calories: 120; Fat: 10g; Phosphorus: 10mg; Potassium: 107mg; Sodium: 31mg; Carbohydrates: 5g; Protein: 1.2g.

Cashew and Almond Butter

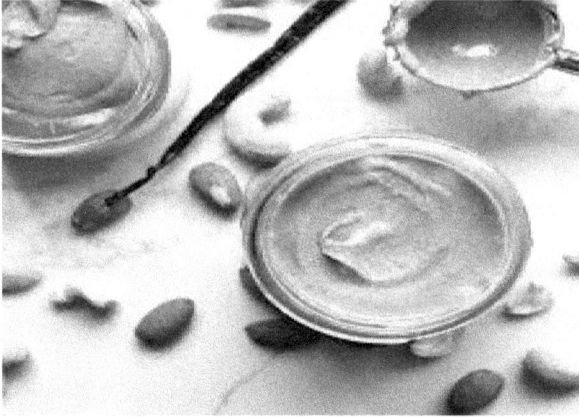

Preparation Time: 5 minutes

Cooking Time: Nil

Serving: 2

INGREDIENTS:

- o 1 cup almonds; blanched
- o 1/3 cup cashew nuts
- o 2 tablespoons coconut oil
- o Salt as needed
- o ½ teaspoon cinnamon

DIRECTIONS:

1) Preheat your oven to 350°F.
2) Bake almonds and cashews for 12 minutes.
3) Let them cool.
4) Transfer to a food processor and add remaining ingredients.
5) Add oil and keep blending until smooth.
6) Serve and enjoy!

NUTRITION (Per Serving): Calories: 205; Fat: 19g; Phosphorus: 23mg; Potassium: 102mg; Sodium: 20mg; Carbohydrates: g; Protein: 2.8g.

Measurement Conversion Chart

American and British Variances					
Term	Abbreviation	Nationality	Dry or liquid	Metric equivalent	Equivalent in context
cup	c., C.		usually liquid	237 milliliters	16 tablespoons or 8 ounces
ounce	fl oz, fl. oz.	American	liquid only	29.57 milliliters	
		British	either	28.41 milliliters	
gallon	gal.	American	liquid only	3.785 liters	4 quarts
		British	either	4.546 liters	4 quarts
inch	in, in.			2.54 centimeters	
ounce	oz, oz.	American	dry	28.35 grams	1/16 pound
			liquid	see OUNCE	see OUNCE
pint	p., pt.	American	liquid	0.473 liter	1/8 gallon or 16 ounces
			dry	0.551 liter	1/2 quart
		British	either	0.568 liter	
pound	lb.		dry	453.592 grams	16 ounces
Quart	q., qt, qt.	American	liquid	0.946 liter	1/4 gallon or 32 ounces
			dry	1.101 liters	2 pints
		British	either	1.136 liters	
Teaspoon	t., tsp., tsp		either	about 5 milliliters	1/3 tablespoon
Tablespoon	T., tbs., tbsp.		either	about 15 milliliters	3 teaspoons or 1/2 ounce

Volume (Liquid)

American Standard (Cups & Quarts)	American Standard (Ounces)	Metric (Milliliters & Liters)
2 tbsp.	1 fl. oz.	30 ml
1/4 cup	2 fl. oz.	60 ml
1/2 cup	4 fl. oz.	125 ml
1 cup	8 fl. oz.	250 ml
1 1/2 cups	12 fl. oz.	375 ml
2 cups or 1 pint	16 fl. oz.	500 ml
4 cups or 1 quart	32 fl. oz.	1000 ml or 1 liter
1 gallon	128 fl. oz.	4 liters

Volume (Dry)

American Standard	Metric
1/8 teaspoon	5 ml
1/4 teaspoon	1 ml
1/2 teaspoon	2 ml
3/4 teaspoon	4 ml
1 teaspoon	5 ml
1 tablespoon	15 ml
1/4 cup	59 ml
1/3 cup	79 ml
1/2 cup	118 ml
2/3 cup	158 ml
3/4 cup	177 ml
1 cup	225 ml
2 cups or 1 pint	450 ml
3 cups	675 ml
4 cups or 1 quart	1 liter
1/2 gallon	2 liters
1 gallon	4 liters

Dry Measure Equivalents

3 teaspoons	1 tablespoon	1/2 ounce	14.3 grams
2 tablespoons	1/8 cup	1 ounce	28.3 grams
4 tablespoons	1/4 cup	2 ounces	56.7 grams
5 1/3 tablespoons	1/3 cup	2.6 ounces	75.6 grams
8 tablespoons	1/2 cup	4 ounces	113.4 grams
12 tablespoons	3/4 cup	6 ounces	.375 pound
32 tablespoons	2 cups	16 ounces	1 pound

Oven Temperatures

American Standard	Metric
250° F	130° C
300° F	150° C
350° F	180° C
400° F	200° C
450° F	230° C

Weight (Mass)

American Standard (Ounces)	Metric (Grams)
1/2 ounce	15 grams
1 ounce	30 grams
3 ounces	85 grams
3.75 ounces	100 grams
4 ounces	115 grams
8 ounces	225 grams
12 ounces	340 grams
16 ounces or 1 pound	450 grams

www.ingramcontent.com/pod-product-compliance
Lightning Source LLC
Chambersburg PA
CBHW050744030426
42336CB00012B/1644